ON YOUR FEET

A practicing podiatrist tells you how to maintain foot health and comfort from infancy to old age.

W9-CJM-619

ON YOUR FEET

A practicing podiatrist tells you how to maintain foot health and comfort from infancy to old age.

Elizabeth H. Roberts, D.P.M.

Designed and Illustrated by Donald Breter

Rodale Press, Book Division
Emmaus, Pa., 18049

Copyright © 1975, 1980 by Elizabeth Roberts

Chapter 13 revised

All rights reserved. No part of this publication may
be reproduced or transmitted in any form or by any
means, electronic or mechanical, including photocopy,
recording, or any information storage and retrieval
system, without the written permission of the
publisher.

Printed in the United States of America on recycled paper,
containing a high percentage of de-inked fiber.

Library of Congress Cataloging in Publication Data

Roberts, Elizabeth H
    On your feet.

    Includes index.
    1. Foot—Care and hygiene. 2. Foot—Diseases.
I. Title. [DNLM: 1. Podiatry—Popular works. WE890
R6430]
RD563.R56 1980   617'.585052   79-27498
ISBN 0-87857-099-3 hardcover
ISBN 0-87857-292-9 paperback

  4 6 8 10 9 7 5 3   hardcover

2 4 6 8 10 9 7 5 3 1 paperback

Dedication

To

Nat, my late husband, for his generosity in arranging time for me to write this book and for his unfailing ability to supply the word that had been eluding me

and

Judy, my daughter, without whose urging this book would not have been undertaken and without whose interest it would not have been completed.

Acknowledgments

In 1974 when I first wrote this book, I thanked several people, most of them authorities in their fields, for their generosity in sharing with me both their knowledge and their time.

I spoke of my gratitude to Miss Margaret McElderry, Dr. Malcolm Jacobson, Mrs. Fella Friede, Dr. Herman Sonderling, Dr. Benjamin Kauth, Mr. Donald Breter, Mrs. Helen Breter, Miss Sheila Netz, who is now Mrs. Bogdan Sennenbrot, Mr. Gilbert Hollander, Dr. Norman Klombers, Dr. Richard O. Schuster, Dr. Seymour C. Frank, and Dr. Alexander Fisher. Another whom I thanked was Mr. Charles Gerras, my editor, who still listens, generally expedites, and consistently speaks with wisdom.

They and others, too, have helped me in completely rewriting, with extensive additions, the chapter on sports in this edition.

I should like to elaborate on just how helpful each of these additional people has been, but space permits only a listing of their names. I, however, shall remember how special each has been.

They are Dr. Harvey Strauss, Dr. Charles Ross, Dr. Sheldon Langer, Dr. Justin Wernick, Dr. Stuart E. Kirshenbaum, Dr. Jack Gorman, Dr. Bernard Helfand, Dr. Ralph Mazer, Mr. Louis Buttell, and Miss Dian Sutherland.

A very special message of gratitude goes to my daughter, who back in 1974 was Miss Judith N. Wasserheit and who today is Judith N. Wasserheit, M.D. My gratitude is not only for her incisive editing of everything I write, but for the sincerity of interest and warmth of love that we share.

Since that original writing in 1974, *On Your Feet* has had quite a history in its own right—three printings in the first year, a mass paperback edition, and— about this I am most pleased—it was chosen by the Library of Congress to be put on tape cassettes for the blind.

Elizabeth H. Roberts

October 1979

Preface

As president of the Long Island University, College of Podiatry, I had the opportunity to learn the capabilities of the author of this book as a student in our college and as an interne in our clinics.

Dr. Elizabeth H. Roberts was graduated cum laude from Long Island University College of Podiatry. For many years she lectured on anatomy of the foot and leg. This set the stage for her to keep abreast of the most current concepts in diagnosis and therapeutics in the practice of Podiatric Medicine. Her dedication to her profession is evidenced by her service on the staff of the Foot Clinics of New York, by her having established the Diabetic Foot Clinic at the New York Infirmary and by her appointment to the courtesy staff of the Midtown Hospital.

At this writing Dr. Roberts is Professor Emeritus at the New York College of Podiatric Medicine and a Fellow of the Academy of Podiatric Medicine. Her most recent achievement is her appointment by the Board of Regents of the State of New York to the State Board for Podiatry. She is the author of a textbook and has had many articles published in professional journals and lay magazines. In addition to lecturing to scientific and lay groups, she appears on radio and television programs dealing with podiatric topics.

Dr. Roberts has a daughter, Judy, who is now attending Harvard Medical School. In watching Judy grow, she has had the opportunity to observe at close range the development of coordination and interplay of the feet with other parts of the body. Dr. Roberts is uniquely qualified to serve as your consultant in the care of your feet.

The ability to recognize symptoms gives you the opportunity to arrest the development of abnormalities before they progress beyond functional control.

On Your Feet stresses symptoms highlighted by the many illustrations throughout the book. Guidance is given as to when and how and where to seek professional advice.

Herman Sonderling, D.P.M., Hon. D.Sc.
President Emeritus
New York College of Podiatric Medicine
October 1974

Contents

Chapter **1**

How Old Do You Walk?

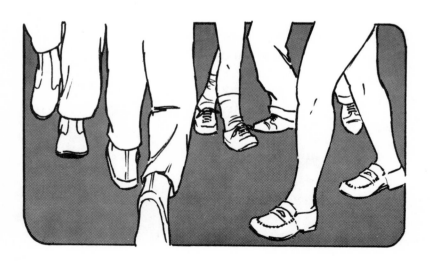

It's a game I play.

Try it some time when you're walking down a busy street. Watch someone walking in front of you, someone whose face you can't see. Then guess that person's age. Next maneuver your way abreast of him and try to verify your guess by glancing at his face and general appearance.

I bet you'll be wrong just as often as I am. Of course, I, as a podiatrist, actually enjoy my errors in judgment —because each error is proof that a bad gait can add years to one's appearance by its awkwardness, its apparent painfulness, its lack of rhythm, its "stepping-on-hot-coals" hesitancy. It is equal proof that a good gait can subtract years from one's appearance by its spring, its stride, its rhythm, its ease.

You can't look young if you clomp along as though not a joint in your body is capable of motion. The twenty-year old who stumbles along with obvious pain looks years older than the sixty-year-old who swings along with evident ease.

Many factors enter into your ability or inability to

walk young. A prime factor, of course, is your own genes—the kind of body with which you started.

We all know the person who will recall, with either resentment or resignation, "My father had a hammertoe just like mine—same foot, same toe!" or, "My mother was always complaining about her bunions."

It's great to have parents on whom you can blame even your foot problems, but most foot conditions are *not* inherited. What is inherited is a body with certain potentials for development, normal and abnormal. Thus, some bodies will develop hammertoes more readily than others, just as some bodies will develop bunions more readily than others. Because of their genes some people tend to develop a muscular imbalance of their feet and legs; others develop circulatory problems or arthritis or other generalized body conditions that are manifested in their feet. Fortunately, much can be done today to prevent or to ameliorate these difficulties.

While your genes determine your body's potential for development—desirable or undesirable, what you do with your body is another consideration. If the body belongs to a Guatemalan Indian, walking barefoot on soft soil, the feet will develop differently from those of an equally healthy New York businesswoman, walking in confining shoes in an office during the day, standing in confining shoes in a subway car at the end of the working day, stopping to do her marketing on the way home and then standing to prepare dinner and to do the necessary household chores. Obviously there is a great differential in both stress and fatigue factors.

I have often been told by patients, particularly by women who do not go to business, that they had had

2

no awareness of foot problems until they moved from the suburbs to the city. The mode of dress—including shoes—is more informal in the suburbs. Sneakers or thongs are acceptable for daytime use. The woman of comparable social status, living in the city, spends her day in more constricting shoes, in keeping with her more formal attire.

In the suburbs one gets into an automobile to go from place to place, even if the distance is short. In a city such as New York one walks short distances. One uses public transportation—buses, subways, taxis. And one stands waiting for any one of them. Yes, in the city you walk and walk and stand and stand! If you can't walk young and stand young, you're in trouble.

Occupation is another point of difference in the way people use their bodies. The demands on the body of a fashion model in high heels are different from the demands on the body of a nurse in regulation shoes. The truckdriver making deliveries, jumping down from the truck many times a day, uses his body differently from the way the dentist uses his, whether or not the latter stands to treat his patients.

Obviously you can't consider your feet separately from the rest of your body. One major highlight about your feet and the care of your feet is evident:

YOU CANNOT HAVE A FOOT PROBLEM WITH- OUT HAVING THAT PROBLEM REFLECTED IN OTHER PARTS OF YOUR BODY.

If your foot posture is incorrect, the alignment of your entire body structure above your feet must be incorrect. (I often comment to patients that the Leaning Tower of Pisa is leaning not because of the structure, but because of the foundation.) As a result of this

3

interdependence of the feet and the structures above them, many patients complaining of lower back pains are referred by their general practitioners or by their internists to podiatrists. Lower back pains may come from many causes, but high on the list is faulty foot function.

A corollary to the fact that you cannot have a foot problem without having that problem reflected in other parts of your body is:

MANY PROBLEMS IN OTHER PARTS OF YOUR BODY WILL AFFECT PROPER FOOT FUNCTION.

This, in turn, will aggravate the original problem. A good example is difficulty with the right knee, which eventually leads to improper use of the right foot, thus causing greater stress on the right knee! Furthermore, since the right foot and leg are not functioning at an optimum level, the left foot and leg will be subject to excessive weight-bearing demands which may result in difficulties on the left side.

We must, therefore, accept still a third fact:

TREATMENT OF THE FEET TO IMPROVE COMFORT AND FUNCTION WILL FAVORABLY AFFECT OTHER PARTS OF THE BODY.

Frequently this will minimize or eliminate such symptoms as fatigue and leg cramping.

Never entertain the fallacious old saw, "I'm too old to do anything about it!" Whether you're seventeen or seventy, don't resign yourself to foot discomfort or to fatigue without at least trying to have it eliminated. There is sheer defeat in the philosophy that, "I'm not as young as I once was. I can't expect to get around the way I used to." Even if you can't get around as you did thirty years ago, the chances are good that with proper podiatric care you can walk with greater comfort and with less fatigue than you experience now.

Although we're discussing foot care, let me urge you not to accept any body disability on the basis of "I'm not as young as I once was." Whether the symptoms are in your feet or in any other part of your body, it is probable that you can feel better—and younger —if you have proper medical attention. It is wasteful of years of your life to settle for less than your body can offer you!

Make the most of what you have and you'll feel younger—and you'll walk younger!

Chapter **2**

Your Feet Are Part
of Your Body

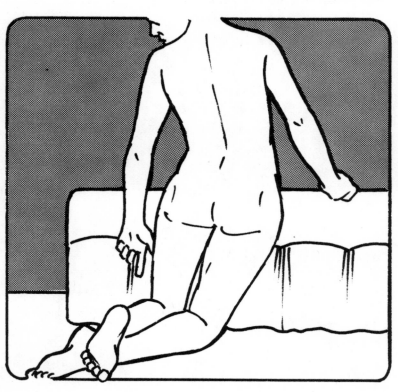

Many of us speak of our feet as though they were attached in some mysterious way—perhaps by wires —to the rest of the body, but had no real effect on the body, and as though the body had no real effect on the feet.

Patients who come to me with a corn are amazed when I ask, "Have you any lower back pain?"

Often the answer is, "I sure have, but what has that to do with my corn?"

Every once in awhile a patient will resent being asked details of his general health. "It's just my feet that are bothering me."

I have *almost* become accustomed to the amazement of these people when I explain that a deficiency in one part of the body will affect other parts of the body— and that the feet are part of the body. For example, an arterial incident in the brain or an injury to the spinal cord may paralyze the arm, the leg or both.

All the parts of your body are supplied by the blood of one circulatory system, by the interplay of one muscular system, by the innervation of one neurologic system.

Your feet are a magnificently well-engineered part of your body. They carry the weight of your entire body. They help to hold your body in a stationary, upright position. They coordinate to maintain your body's balance as you walk. They allow you to accelerate your pace as you run. They have the precision that permits you to leave the ground completely and return in an upright position as you jump.

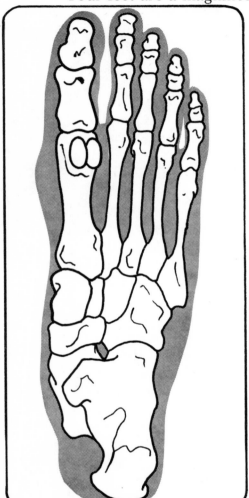

Each of your feet is generally described as having twenty-six bones. Actually there are twenty-eight bones in each foot. Twenty-six of them articulate with one or more adjacent bones. Two small round bones, called sesamoid bones, are anchored in the tendons at the bottom of your foot behind the great toe.

Some people have additional small sesamoid bones. These are called supernumerary sesamoids and usually are found in identical places in each foot. People with supernumerary sesamoids in the feet will often reveal, on x-ray examination, supernumerary bones in other parts of the body. These small bones denote no abnormality, simply having occurred in the normal development of these individuals. My patients, however, always feel a certain distinction in having a few extra bones!

We are most interested in the twenty-six primary bones in each of your feet. Fourteen of the twenty-six are in your toes—three in each of the smaller toes and two in the great toe.

The great toe is the longest in most feet, but it is thoroughly normal for the second toe (next to the great toe) or even the third toe to be longer than the great toe. While it is anatomically normal, it certainly can be a shoe-fitting problem!

The longitudinal arch is the concave area extending from the heel to the ball on the inner side of the foot. If you want to determine whether your longitudinal arch is as high as it should be, don't depend on wet footprints in the sand. 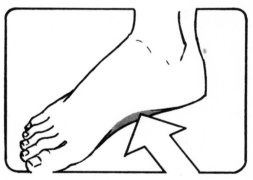 Stand as you usually do. Have someone draw a line from the midpoint of your knee to the midpoint of your leg below the knee and continue it down to your foot. If the line is perpendicular to the surface on which you're standing, with no deviation to the side of your foot, your longitudinal arch is at its norm.

Some people normally have very low or flat longitudinal arches. The person who was born with a flat arch is said to have a congenital flatfoot. The midline

9

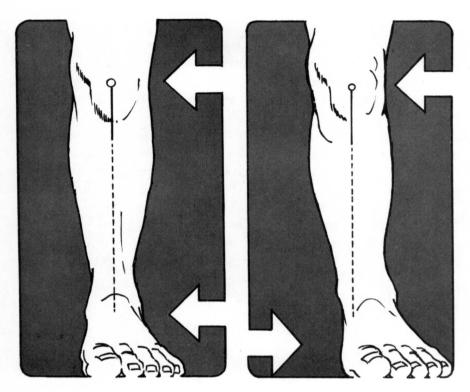

of his knee and of his leg will form a line perpendicular to the floor in spite of his arch being completely flat. The person who has an acquired flatfoot, and for whom it is an abnormality, will have the line from the midpoint of his knee to the midpoint of his leg going off to the side of his foot.

The congenital flatfoot may not be graceful, but it is extremely serviceable. The armed forces learned this after having rejected all flatfooted men during World War I. By World War II men with congenital flatfeet were accepted, because it was now understood that theirs were feet least likely to suffer under the stress of long marches.

10

The so-called metatarsal arch is at the ball of your foot. It is more accurate to speak of the metatarsal area, since it is generally agreed that the bones in the ball of the foot do not form an arch.

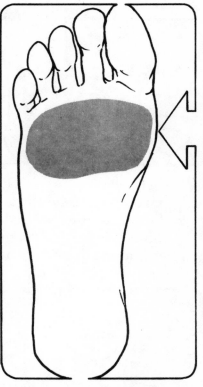

Bones are held in relationship to each other by ligaments, which are bands of strong white fibers. The point of junction between ar-

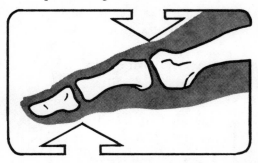

ticulating bones is known as a joint. In the foot all the joints are movable, making possible varied positions. There are joints in the body that are not movable, as in the skull. Think what rattle-brains we would be if the joints in our skulls permitted the bones to move hither and yon!

The ability to stand, to walk, to run, to dance, to skate and to perform the other multifarious activities in which we participate, without giving thought to how they are accomplished, depends on many factors in addition to the bones, the ligaments and the joints.

Muscles, thirteen of them in your leg and twenty of them in your foot, control both the extent and the

11

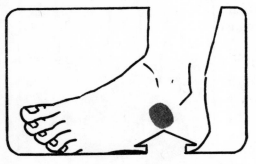

direction of the motion of your foot. Only one of these muscles, the *extensor brevis digitorum,* is on the top surface of your foot. It is just in front of the ankle, toward the outer side. In many feet it appears as a well-defined prominence. For this reason some people mistake this muscle for a swelling. Some of them are relieved to be assured that there's no abnormality; others seem downright disappointed at having nothing more dramatic than a muscle that belongs there anyway!

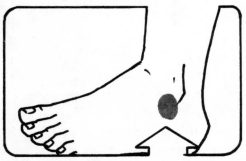

Many women in their forties and fifties develop a fat pad just below and in front of the outer side of the ankle. This, too, is often mistaken for a swelling. A good test for whether or not it is a swelling is to check if the area changes in size. Is it smaller in the morning? Is it larger after a day on your feet? A swelling will change in size; a fat pad will not.

When you stand on your toes, two of the muscles in the back of your leg, the *gastrocnemius* and the *soleus,* contract, pulling on a tendon, and thus raising your heel. Girl-watchers, admiring a pair of shapely legs, are seldom aware that this shapeliness is probably the overdevelopment of these muscles resulting from the overuse of high heels—pretty much the equivalent of standing constantly on one's toes. They also don't know that these shapely legs might no longer be able to wear low heels because the muscles have shortened. How could they guess that these shapely legs might be so painful in walking barefoot that the lady in question always walks on her tiptoes until she gets into her high-heeled shoes?

The tendon which goes from these muscles to the heel is called the *tendo-Achilles.* You may recall that Achilles was the mightiest of the Greek warriors in the Trojan War. His mother, Thetis, with commendable maternal intent, dipped the baby, Achilles, into the River Styx in an attempt to make him immortal. With understandable maternal concern she grasped him so as not to lose him. She grasped him by his heel—the only part not immersed in the river and, therefore, the only part to remain vulnerable. Thus, this mightiest of warriors was killed by a mortal wound—in his heel. Never let it be said that anatomists, in selecting their nomenclature, have neither a knowledge of the classics nor a sense of humor!

Both muscles and bones have a blood supply, which is the source of their nourishment. Without an adequate blood supply there is death of tissue, as in gangrene. The lower extremity—the foot and the leg—is the area most frequently involved in poor circulation and consequent therapy as dramatic as amputation. The upper extremity—the hand and the arm—enjoy, for the most part, better circulation.

Just as you have a pulse in your wrist, you normally have two pulses that are palpable in the foot. One, the *dorsalis pedis* pulse, is found on the top of the foot on

13

a line between the great toe and the second toe. The other, the *posterior tibial* pulse, is found be-

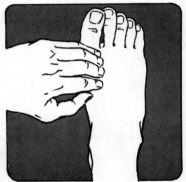
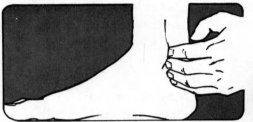

hind the bone on the inner side of the ankle. These are the two pulses which your doctor will check in examining your feet. If you want to try finding them on your own foot, use just the tips of your four lesser fingers, not your thumb, and don't decide all is lost if you can't feel them. Your automobile may have each part exactly where the manufacturer indicates it should be, but your body was not factory specified. The pulse may be a little to the right or a little to the left, a little above or a little below where most people have it. There may be enough fatty tissue covering it that it's not readily palpable. When you do palpate a pulse, you're feeling the contraction and expansion of an artery in time with the heartbeat.

Since your feet are part of your body, they are subject to circulation problems that might occur in other parts of your body. An arterial block or hardening of the arteries, for example, may result in insufficient blood reaching the legs and feet. Another example is anemia, as a result of which the blood does not adequately nourish the parts it supplies. On the other hand, failure of your foot and leg to function at an optimum may create interference with the proper re-

14

turn of blood to the rest of the body. Muscles, by their normal action in contracting and relaxing, provide a massaging effect on the blood vessels, helping them to maintain normal passage of blood.

If you look carefully at the top of your foot, you'll see a bluish arc just behind your toes. The arc continues back along the foot. On most feet it seems to disappear in front of the ankle. On some feet it is far 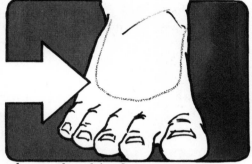 more prominent than on others, the thin foot generally demonstrating it best. If you've found the arc on your own foot, you're looking at veins, the vessels through which blood is returned from the foot to the rest of the body. If you haven't found it, don't fret. You're not without veins; those particular veins are just not as visible in your foot as they are in some others.

Veins of the lower extremities are found, for the most part, in a fascinating arrangement of two sets, one superficial and one deep. Generally, when your doctor speaks of varicose veins, he's referring to a condition of the superficial veins in which the tiny valves within the veins are not capable of maintaining the flow of blood against gravity up to the veins of the rest of the body. Before the doctor treats varicose veins, he usually asks the patient to go through various tests, like elevating the leg for a specific period and then lowering it, by way of determining whether the deep veins are capable of taking on the additional job of the superficial vessels. This is essential, since treatment for varicose veins, regardless of the nature of treatment, generally has as its goal the elimination of the functioning of the varicosed veins.

Capillaries are tiny vessels which, in the foot and leg, as in any other part of the body, connect the arteries with the veins.

The nerves that go to the foot and the leg come from the spinal cord at the lower part of the back—the lumbar and the sacral regions. Good innervation from the spinal cord to the foot and leg is essential for efficient muscle function to initiate and maintain walking, running, standing or more intricate movements, such as bowling or dancing. It is essential, too, for accurate sensation like touch, pain and position.

I truly wish that everyone could have the privilege of watching a dissection of a human cadaver to see the magnificent interlacing of blood vessels—arteries, veins and capillaries—and of nerves extending throughout the body with the precision of an unbelievably complicated master plan.

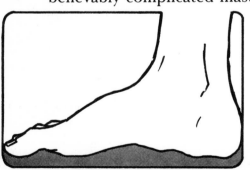 Your foot functions in two distinct, but complementary, ways. It must have all the looseness and adaptability of a bean bag so that it can conform to any type of surface, even or uneven, while still holding the upright position of your leg and of the rest of your body. The movable joints of the foot implement this phase of weight bearing, emphasizing the importance of retaining adequate joint spaces.

16

Secondly, this "bean bag" must have the capacity to become a rigid unit to lift your body and to step forward.

While we define a *range* of normal gait, studies have proven that the gait pattern of your right foot is not identical with that of your left. There is no point in normal gait when the total foot is flat on the ground. In optimum walking the toes point

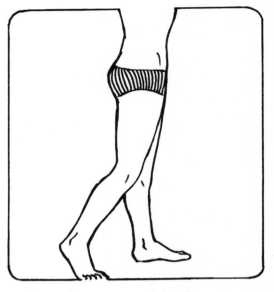

straight ahead. The first point of contact with the ground is that of the heel. The weight is then carried along the outer border of the foot to the ball, across the ball to the great toe.

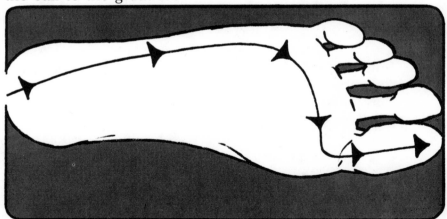

You might look at the sole of a pair of your shoes to check your own gait. Fairly new shoes are often

17

more revealing than older ones. Ideally the marks of wear should include the outer rim of the shoes, but not the entire inner rim. Frequently shoes will show only a small area of weight bearing in the center of the sole because the gait is so abnormal that there is ground contact with just a fraction of the shoe.

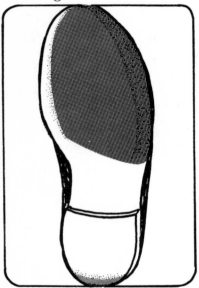 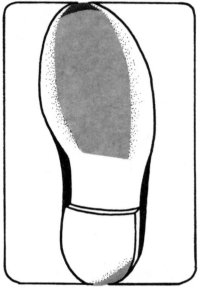

There are great differences in normal gait, depending on both physical and psychological factors. Ectomorphic people, the slender, linear type, generally have a more agile gait than do endomorphic people. The endomorph has the heavier, stocky body, with a slower, more plodding gait. The mesomorph is the big-boned, athletic type who probably achieves the most efficient type of gait.

Psychological factors are transmitted to gait. The strut of the bully is very distinct from the mincing steps of Mr. Milquetoast.

Walking, while a lower extremity function, brings

18

into play other parts of the body. Dr. M. Beckett Howorth described this well in "The Art and Technique of Walking" (*Consumer Bulletin,* April, 1973):

. . . the trunk muscles—abdominal, flank, back, and chest —contract to hold the trunk erect and to swing the leg. The opposite arm swings forward with the leg by contraction of the shoulder and hip flexors, and the wrist extensors, and back by the action of their antagonists.

The diaphragm, abdominal muscles, and muscles of the ribs expand the chest and lungs as we breathe . . .

The action of the muscles is dependent on the circulation, the heart, the lungs, and the nerves. Fuel for muscle action is brought by the arteries, and waste products are carried away by the veins, with the heart acting as the pump for the circulation of blood. The blood flows through the lungs, where carbon dioxide is eliminated, and oxygen for combustion acquired, and through the liver, where fuel, stored from the digestive tract, is obtained.

The nerves carry the stimuli for contraction to the muscle, and the sense of position to the central nervous system. Thus most of the muscles, and most of the organs and tissues, participate in the simple act of walking.

Standing is far more tiring than walking. One of the most difficult jobs, physically, is that of the elevator operator who must stand hour upon hour with a minimum of change in position. There is constant demand on the same muscles, in contrast to walking where first one set of muscles, and then another, is brought into play. That is the reason standing in a crowd to watch a parade is synonymous with fidgeting from one foot to another.

There is one trick you might remember the next time you watch a parade, or wait for a train on a crowded station, or are jammed into less than human space on a subway, or wait in a queue for a gift wrapping in a department store. Stand on the outer bor-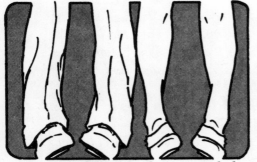ders of your feet with your feet pointing straight ahead. Be sure you're rolled way over to the outer edges and be sure the toes point straight ahead. You may not look glamorous, but you'll be much more comfortable for a much longer period. And who can see your feet in a crowd?

It is because of the muscular interplay that it is easiest and most efficient to arise from a sitting position by placing one or both feet under the chair and then tilting the body forward.

Thus, with both intricacy and logic the rest of your body contributes to and, at the same time, is dependent on the functioning of your feet.

Chapter **3**

When It All Begins

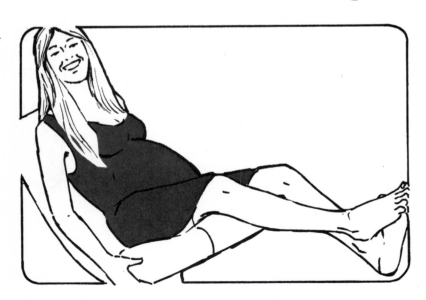

Nature has a timetable for development long before your baby is born.

Normally each part of the body develops at a specific time. By the sixth week of fetal life the foot and leg have begun to form. There follows a rate of growth so rapid that the foot length doubles during the fourth month before birth.

At birth the average foot length is three to three and a quarter inches. (The average size of the adult woman's foot is eight inches, of the adult man's foot eleven inches.) According to Dr. Herman Tax, a New York podiatrist and author of the textbook, *Podo Pediatrics, The Care of Children's Feet,* it takes four years to double the length of the foot at birth and eight years to double the length of the foot at six months.

At birth the bones are not fully formed. There is cartilage between portions of bone. As a result, an x-ray of a baby's foot differs from that of an adult not only in size, but also in the appearance of the bones. There seem to be more bones in the baby's and child's foot because all of these cartilaginous areas do not

23

become bone tissue until as late as the eighteenth to twenty-second year.

Soon after birth your doctor examines your baby to determine whether all is normal.

Immediately after you bring your baby home from the hospital, friends and relatives gather to gaze with admiration. And thus it should be. Just because there are babies being born every day is no reason to forget the sheer wonderment of each new baby.

You, the mother, have the joy of feeling your baby's growth and movement within your body. You also have the responsibility for maintaining your own health and for following a way of life that will give to your baby the optimum chance to be born normal and vigorous.

You may have some periods of downright discomfort, compensated for only by the knowledge that pregnancy is a period of creativity, not of pathology. During pregnancy foot and leg fatigue sometimes becomes extreme. Many women experience a feeling of heaviness of the legs. Some complain of acute leg cramping. Varicose veins often become apparent. It's sometimes difficult to philosophize that this is a small price to pay for the miracle of childbearing. But small price or no, it does help to remember that this cramping, heaviness and fatigue will disappear when your baby is born. In many instances the varicose veins also disappear.

The condition of your feet during pregnancy can affect not only your comfort, but the well-being of your baby. If you're walking incorrectly, there is a distortion in the position of your legs, of your knees, of your thighs, and of your pelvis. You owe your baby as much space as possible for development within you.

24

Don't diminish that space by going through a pregnancy without professional care for your feet.

This, incidentally, is a matter I always discuss with my newly married female patients. Achieving good foot function well in advance of a pregnancy is that much in your favor!

Remember, too, that your feet and legs will be carrying the weight of your baby. Your obstetrician will urge you to guard your weight gain during these months. Your podiatrist will agree wholeheartedly.

Not only will faulty standing and walking throw the rest of your body out of proper alignment, but any foot pain will cause you automatically to pull away from the painful area. A corn or a callus, an ingrown nail, a wart, a crack between your toes—any painful abnormality—will make you walk off kilter. Even if you don't mind the heroics of unnecessary pain, remember that baby inside you.

Pain also makes for instability in walking, increasing the chance of falling. And if ever you want to be sure not to fall, it's during pregnancy.

Walking is a must for a pregnant woman, and thus shoes are of prime importance. Your shoes should provide a firm walking surface. They should have the lowest, broadest heel *that is comfortable for you.* If, for several years, you have consistently worn two-inch heels, you probably can't wear a low heel comfortably. The muscles in the back of your legs have shortened and it would be not only uncomfortable, but actually dangerous, for you suddenly to wear a low heel. You should wear the lowest, broadest heel *that you can comfortably tolerate.*

It is a fact of shoe design that generally the higher the heel, the narrower the heel and the more pointed the toe. This thrusts your foot forward, and makes for cramped toes. If you can't wear a low heel early in your pregnancy, buy a shoe with a heel only one lift lower than you ordinarily wear. After three weeks, remove one lift from that heel. A lift is a quarter of an inch. One lift can be removed from any heel without changing the tilt of the shoe. (One lift can also be added to any heel without changing the contour of the shoe, but this is not the time for lift adding!)

If the heel is still high, after three weeks of wearing that shoe with the lift change, buy another with a heel still one lift lower than that which you are now discarding. Thus, in gradual stages, early in your pregnancy, you can become accustomed to a lower, broader heel.

Fortunately, and this is said with a salute to our young people who seek for themselves a natural comfort, most of the young mothers of today are accustomed to slacks and low heels. They don't have to worry about shortened calf muscles.

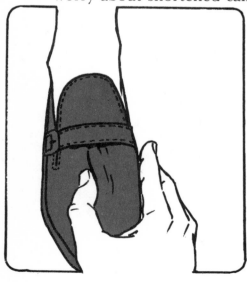

Since your feet will probably swell while you're pregnant—and all the more in warm weather—shoes must allow for that swelling. This doesn't mean getting a shoe too big for safety. While there should be a snug heel fit, the leather across the top of the shoe should be loose enough to ripple as a finger is rolled across it. It is a fact, however, that perhaps eighty percent of the women I see in my office have, through the years, been consistently fitted with shoes too small for them. There should be adequate depth from the top of the shoe to the sole to avoid pressure on your toes.

During pregnancy don't wear plastic, patent leather or reptile shoes. They lack porosity and flexibility. You don't have to get a matronly type of shoe. A soft lightweight leather, suede or fabric in a college girl type of oxford is most desirable.

Rubber heel lifts are safer than leather. Above all, avoid the synthetic lifts because they are frequently slippery. It's worth changing the lifts even on a brand new pair of shoes if they aren't rubber. Be sure, too, that you don't let your heels become run-down. This is, in itself, a factor of instability.

For a "scotch-and-soda" shoe that every about-to-be mother should have for those dress-up occasions, you might get a low heeled step-in, but do keep it for dress-up!

Don't depend on mules or flimsy slippers when you're working at home. You might fall!

Walking barefoot at the beach, on soft ground, or even on a high pile rug is great exercise.

Now, fortified with all this information, sally forth on your daily walks with comfort and with enjoyment.

You may find that you're developing varicose veins. Whether or not they are to be treated during pregnancy should be the decision of your obstetrician. Maintaining good foot function, however, helps to maintain circulation in your legs.

When you do hold that newly arrived baby in your arms, don't decide that you need no longer care for YOU. Do remember YOU for the sake of your baby.

We live lives far more sophisticated, and perhaps debilitating, than do the women who have their babies in the rice fields and then get right back to work. It takes a minimum of six weeks for your body to restore itself to its pre-pregnancy condition. This is too frequently forgotten these days. The present therapeutic philosophy encourages you to walk very soon after your delivery; the current shortage of hospital beds leads to your being sent home in a minimum number of days. And the scarcity and high cost of household help has you back on full-time housekeeping duty almost at once.

There are some other suggestions that are particularly applicable to you during your pregnancy.

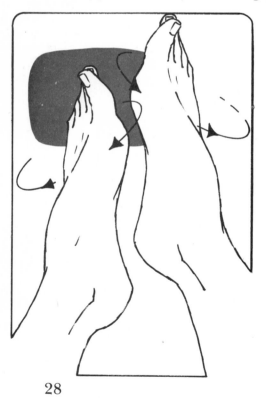

1. As you sit watching television or reading, rotate your feet at your ankles, turning the feet in so that the soles face each other.

2. Avoid walking barefoot in the dark. Don't risk the pain and inconvenience of a fractured toe from stumbling into a piece of furniture.

3. If your feet perspire excessively, ask your podiatrist to suggest a powder.

28

4. As you dress in the morning and undress at night, walk on the outer borders of your feet, pointing your toes straight ahead.

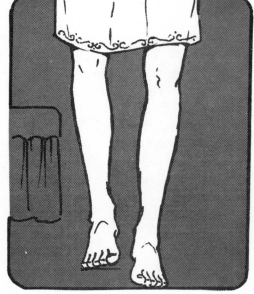

5. Wear hosiery that is amply large for freedom of toe motion. If your obstetrician suggests elasticized hosiery for leg support and for aiding circulation, don't wear the popularly advertised "support" hosiery. It causes compression of the foot, as well as of the leg, sometimes precipitating the development of corns, ulcers or ingrown nails. It may cause uncomfortable constriction of the leg. Buy a pair of toeless (and possibly heelless) surgical hosiery over which you will wear your usual hosiery. These are sold in surgical supply stores, but the best ones are made to measurement by firms specializing in surgical stockings.

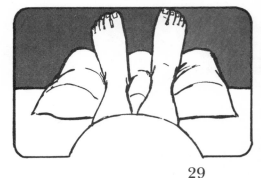

6. Elevating your feet on a pillow at night or during your rest period can add to your comfort and decrease swelling and cramping.

29

7. Don't wear circular garters. They impede the circulation of the leg. If the garter is tight enough to be at all effective, it is too tight for the leg. Today, however, few women wear circular garters. There is need, perhaps, for caution against the ankle or knee socks so frequently worn with slacks. These are held in place by a firmly elasticized band at the top of the hose. Actually this band is a circular garter. Particularly during pregnancy it is imperative to avoid any interference with the circulation of the foot and leg.

Continuing your exercises and staying with proper foot care, which includes comfortable shoes, will help you to be a zestful mother during the pram-pushing and running-after-the-toddler periods!

4

You Can Help Your Baby Develop Healthy Feet

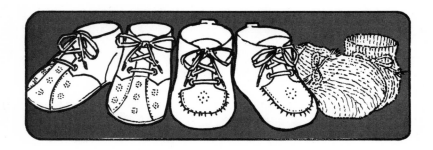

Fast upon the arrival of your baby follows the arrival of gifts of "adorable" little shoes or very tiny handmade booties.

After the thank-you notes have been sent, a display cabinet should be bought for these precious possessions. If you don't want to go to the expense of a display cabinet, then put each pair into a small plastic bag, put them all into a drawer and bring them out only for display purposes.

Don't put them on your baby's feet. It's sad enough that you must wear shoes. Your baby's feet are very malleable; the bones are not completely formed. Give him a chance to wiggle and to stretch and to grow without any impediment or constriction.

The only reason for any foot covering for your baby is the need for warmth. When it's cold, cover his feet with large socks of the cotton, nonstretch variety. These are woven to retain the wide toe space. Another good foot covering when warmth is needed is the baby garment with legs and feet. There are two cautions, however, about either socks or the all-in-one garment:

1. Watch for any shrinkage in washing.

2. Remember that your baby's feet normally grow much more rapidly than any article of clothing will be outworn.

Whatever you use to protect your baby's feet against cold temperatures—and it's important for your baby's general health that his feet be kept warm—remember that it must fit loosely. Just rejoice that the day has not yet arrived for you when your daughter will vie in style with the other girls or your son will insist on too tightly fitting boots!

Your baby's foot is proportionately narrow at the heel and triangular in shape at the sole. While it apparently is good taste to declare that every baby's foot is a thing of beauty, it's sheer tommyrot to assume that all babies are born with perfectly normal feet. All babies are not born with perfectly normal feet, nor are they all born with the potential for normal function. But you can help your baby achieve his own potential by keeping in mind some very basic principles.

1. Blankets that don't allow free motion of the feet and legs can be just as injurious as tight booties 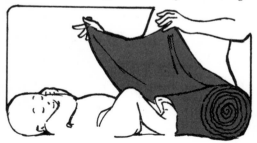 or shoes. If blankets are necessary in spite of warm sleeping garments, tuck them in very loosely over your baby. If you can't resist the temptation to fuss over the covers, place a thick roll of diapers or other bulk at the foot of the crib under the blanket to hold it loosely over your baby's feet.

Apartment dwellers don't always have the advantage home owners have in being able to maintain an even temperature all through the night. I recall that my daughter's pediatrician gave us a simple way of keeping an even temperature—with no concern about blankets. We used an electric room heater regulated by a thermostat. If such a heater is knocked over or tilted, it automatically shuts off. Now, twenty years later, we would not be without the heater in the event of illness in the family.

2. The position of your baby in the crib helps to determine the development of his feet and legs. Don't let him lie constantly on his belly. As a result of this prone position, the toenails are forced against the mattress and are often curved downward against the toes. Fortunately, such nails generally straighten out by the age of four whether they are treated or not.

   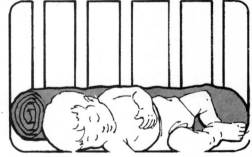

   More important, a constant belly position makes for long-term muscular problems of the feet and legs. Turn your baby periodically as he sleeps. If you want him to stay on his side, use a bolster of diapers or blankets against his back.

3. Nature is great! Nature must be great because one hears so often in discussions about infants' abnormalities, "Nature will take care of it!" Well,

Nature does take care of some problems, but waiting to find out whether Nature will come through with your baby's needs is risky. Give Nature a helping hand and your baby a greater chance for a comfortable, healthy adulthood by consulting your pediatrician, your podiatrist or your orthopedist if you suspect something is wrong.

When you diaper your baby, turn him over and as he lies face down, notice whether the creases

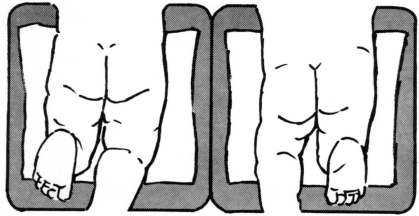

under both the right and left buttocks are even. If there is a discrepancy between the two creases, together with one buttock being flatter and wider than the other, mention it to your pediatrician. He probably has been aware of this. He may feel that, "Nature will take care of it!" You and he may, however, decide that being under his or an orthopedist's supervision or treatment may help Nature.

Nature sometimes corrects overlapping or underlapping toes with which children are born— but, again, don't depend on Nature. Dr. Herman Tax, an outstanding authority on children's feet, states that in about twenty-five percent of infants the second toe overlaps or, less frequently, underlaps the third toe. Consult your pediatrician or your podiatrist.

4. Diapers should not be bulky because they can force the legs into an outward position. Today, however, with the new materials used for diapering, caution is less necessary than formerly. Your doctor may even suggest double diapering to help correct certain hip conditions.

Nature's timetable becomes less rigid as your baby grows, but there is an approximate schedule for such activities as walking, talking or being toilet-trained. These are landmark activities of which parents talk proudly, but which they too often try to accelerate. Your baby can't perform acts for which his body is not adequately developed. Don't expect the impossible.

It's true that the British nanny demands for her charge a potty by the time the baby is three months old. If you're fortunate enough to have a British nanny and she must be coddled, then, by all means, search the shops until you find a cute little potty of which she approves. Plopping your baby on it periodically from three months of age won't hasten sphincter control one bit, but the potty may keep the British nanny in the family—and it makes a stunning planter when you've finally discarded the infant toilet-training idea!

Recognizing and accepting Nature's timetable can save you pointless worry and allow more energy for fun with your baby.

The story is told of a little boy whose parents were distressed because, at two years of age, he was not talking. They took him to a doctor who declared him to be perfectly normal. He assured them the boy would eventually talk, that his vocal chords just weren't ready for this function. When the child was

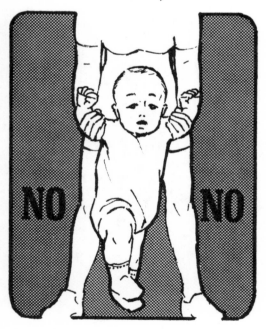

two and a half, his parents again trotted him to the doctor—with the same results. Surely, they thought, theirs must be an abnormal child. Finally, at three years of age, he began to speak. I wonder whether they realized then that their child was indeed unusual. His name was Albert Einstein.

You can do great harm in attempting to hasten Nature's timetable for walking. Your youngster will walk when his body's timetable has allowed for the adequate development of all the muscles necessary for this intricate function.

In the meantime, don't be a dangler. Don't dangle him by his armpits, putting undue strain on his entire musculature. Don't put him into a walker from which his feet can dangle as though he were in high heels. All the dangling in the world won't hasten his walking —and it may impair his muscles. When he's ready to walk, he will! Nature didn't consider the urgency of parental pride in setting up its timetable.

This is the **APPROXIMATE** timetable:

6th month	. . . .	attempts to crawl
8th month	. . . .	attempts to stand
12th month	. . . .	stands well
14th month	. . . .	walks alone
18th month	. . . .	walks fairly well
24th month	. . . .	runs
36th month	. . . .	runs and jumps with real proficiency

The obese child may well take longer to start walking.

Chapter **5**

How You Can Tell Whether Junior Has a Foot Problem

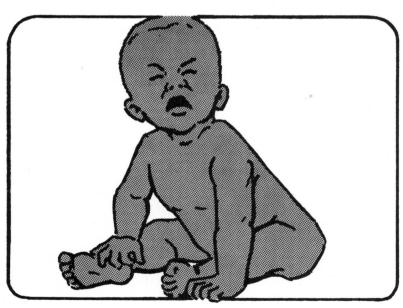

Unless the pain is acute, Junior won't tell you.

And if he's young enough, even if the pain is acute, he may not be able to tell you. His crying will alarm you, not inform you.

Even if he has been talking long enough to communicate the idea of pain, it isn't likely that he's achieved a degree of sophistication to indicate the nature of the pain.

If there is no acute pain, just a discomfort or an ache, he will assume that that is the way he's supposed to feel. This is hardly surprising when you realize that many adults disregard low-grade discomfort, particularly if the onset has been insidious. Adults—grown-up men and women—will tolerate slowly worsening discomfort and slowly decreasing function for years, unnecessarily, just because it is not acute and because it is so easy to forget how one used to feel and move about. If adults rationalize, "I'm getting older. That's what happens!", how can we expect children to know that their bodies should feel or function any other way?

Thus, it becomes the responsibility of parents to be

alert for any symptoms that might indicate foot problems. The significance of oversight or neglect may be far-reaching. Adult foot comfort and function stem from care of the feet from birth. More accurately, we must think of foot comfort and function in relationship to prenatal care since much of the medical thinking today points to various fetal factors as the determinants of future foot health.

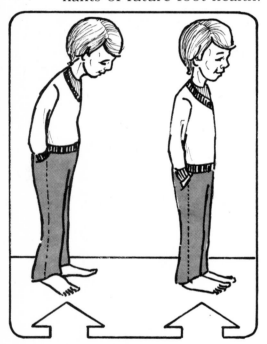

Not only is adult foot health at stake, but the overall development of your child is dependent on proper foot posture. His body posture can't be easy and erect if he doesn't stand and walk properly.

A foot health screening of 8,995 children was conducted in the District of Columbia from 1967 through 1969. Although more than 5,000 of these children were under the age of six, 3,363 had abnormal foot posture. This meant that 37 percent had one strike against them from the very beginning because they could not carry their bodies erect. Moreover, without overall good posture a child's internal organs cannot develop and function at an optimum.

Think for a moment of these figures. More than one third of these 8,995 youngsters, a preponderance of whom were not yet six years old, had postural problems, evident in the feet and gravitating against the normal development of the rest of the body.

I suppose that you have been just as moved as I have been to see a lonely youngster at a playground, standing off and watching the other youngsters running and climbing and jumping. There is something sad and unapproachable about such a youngster, something you don't want for your child. Many of these children get tired more quickly than the others, can't run as fast or are too clumsy to climb and jump with the others. Children are fast to criticize and to taunt.

The child who is left out of games is the child who is left out of parties and all the other peer group events that are so important in establishing self-confidence. A couple of such experiences will quickly teach a child not to expose his inadequacies to his peers. The child whose feet won't meet the tests of his playmates often becomes the teenager who is shy and hesitant to compete or to join in the fun.

Don't expect your child to know that he has a foot problem. You have to investigate for yourself, and if you suspect that the source of the trouble is his feet, don't count on Nature to correct defects. Consult your pediatrician or your podiatrist. Nature should always have a helping hand, even though it be just careful periodic checkups.

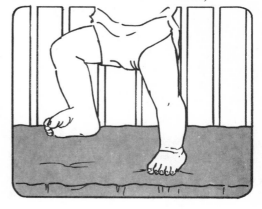

When your offspring starts hauling himself to his feet—with no dangling help from you—it's time to think of new uses for the playpen. A thin mattress generally comes with the playpen. Over that mattress put a soft blanket, large enough to be tucked well under the mattress. Not only does it keep his feet warm, but, as your youngster starts to walk, the blanket provides a soft, grasping surface.

When that great day comes, and you suddenly gasp with delight because Junior has taken his first steps without holding on to a single piece of furniture—well, you'll not notice how he's walking. You'll just gasp. And that's all you're supposed to do at that point. Or perhaps, when that moment is over and his muscles will no longer hold him and he sits smack down on his buttocks, you're supposed to pick him up, kiss him and dash to the telephone to tell Grandma!

But as time goes on, and his muscles develop so that

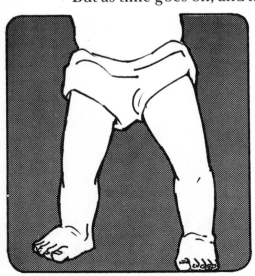

he can maintain his walking, you'll probably notice that he takes a tripod stance, his feet being placed to give him a wide base. At the beginning he will probably hold his arms out for additional stability and will take almost running steps.

This is not the time to look for an arch on your youngster's foot. You won't find any. Unless the foot is exceptionally thin, there is a fat pad under the arch. This fat pad won't disappear until your child is two and one-half or three years old. Even if there is a low arch or practically no arch when the fat pad disappears, this is not necessarily reason for concern. Some of the healthiest feet are those with low or flat arches!

There are, however, various symptoms to which you should be alert. Your alertness is of prime importance, not only because your child won't complain unless the pain is acute, but because too frequently physical examinations are done with the patient stripped except for the shoes and stockings. Somehow feet have been divorced from the rest of the body, even though they are expected to maintain the entire body!

An equally important reason for your alertness is that often much can be seen in watching a child—or anyone else, for that matter—in day-to-day activities. Your doctor can see what's in front of him, can reason cause and effect, but does not have the advantage of following the patient around in his daily activities. Incidentally, try to establish an easy relationship with your doctors in various specialities. Give them some insight into your mode of life and that of your family. It will help them understand what demands are made on your bodies.

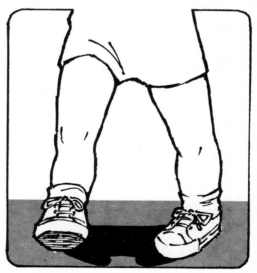

These are some of the symptoms for which you must watch.

1. Does your child toe-in?

    Is this true only when he's walking

barefoot? Is it more marked when shoes are worn? Does he toe-in less in sneakers than in more rigid shoes?

In the infant both inward-toeing and outward-toeing are, according to Dr. Herman Tax, leg rotations that develop stability. But, if inward-toeing persists after your child has been walking long enough to develop stability, consult your

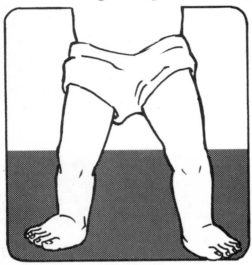

podiatrist. Tell him the circumstances under which you think the gait abnormality exists.

2. Does your child toe-out?

This, after stability in walking has been achieved, is frequently a symptom of weakness of the arch, perhaps the most common of conditions found in children. If weakness of the arch is not treated, it may well cause many adult problems of the feet and of the body in general, problems such as awkward gait, poor posture, excessive fatigue, lower back pain, leg pains and leg cramping.

3. Does your child appear to have knock-knees or bowlegs?

Today nutrition, certainly in this country, has reached a level where diseases such as rickets are seldom found. While your child should most

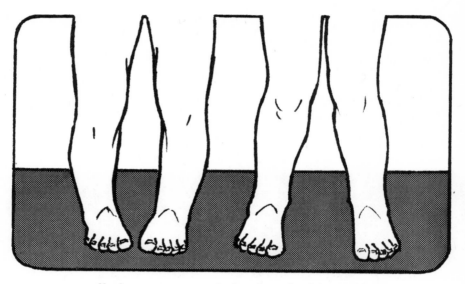

assuredly have a general checkup by his pediatrician, the cause of apparent knee deviation often is improper foot stance and function. It is only through your alertness that your child will be seen by your pediatrician, your orthopedist or your podiatrist.

4. Does your child walk on tiptoes?

   This is often indicative of shortened muscles in the back of the leg. It definitely requires professional consultation.

5. Has your child developed a limp?

   Reasons for a limp are legion.

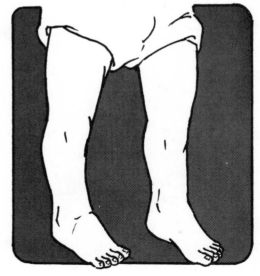

The limp may be the result of an injury that was never mentioned because young people won't gamble on being kept away from playmates for a whole day. This might range from a blister to a cut or an abrasion. (Even playmates won't take precedence over a fracture!)

There may be a limp because of a heel problem that requires professional care over a period of several weeks. A limp might be caused by a wart or a corn or a callus. It might be symptomatic of a neurologic disease or of a difference in the length of the legs.

But, while it is imperative that you have your child examined, don't spend any sleepless nights until you get your appointment. If you must stay awake, try to think whether you know anyone who limps, anyone whom Junior might be imitating! Perhaps Junior knows someone you don't know, someone whose limp appears to be a mighty intriguing abnormality.

Then there is the "ten day limp," a term coined by Dr. Tax to describe a child's limp for which no pathology is found and which generally lasts ten days, at the end of which time it promptly disappears.

Don't, in any event, take upon yourself the diagnosis! Just don't fret in the meantime.

6. Does your child have any small growth on his feet?

    If it is a corn or a callus, your podiatrist will look for the condition that is causing the growth.

Remember that *corns and callus are not conditions; they are symptoms of some underlying condition.*

And is that corn a corn? If you insist on being a diagnostician, are you sure that corn isn't a wart? Countless are the children's feet I have seen with a parent's opening remark, "Amy has a corn." The corn was a wart. Countless are the children's feet I have seen with a parent's opening remark, "Peter has a wart." The wart was a corn.

Medically, a wart is called a *verruca.* When it appears on the bottom of the foot, it is known as a *plantar verruca,* not because it has any relationship to Planters Peanuts or because it was planted there, but because the bottom of the foot is the plantar surface of the foot. A wart, or *verruca,* is a benign tumor, sometimes caused by a virus, frequently found on the feet of children and teenagers, and generally easily differentiated by a podiatrist from a corn.

Warts require treatment because they readily increase in number, sometimes appearing on the hands. Your youngster with a wart should not share a bathmat, socks, slippers or anything that is porous with anyone else for fear of infecting that person. Nonporous surfaces, such as the porcelain of a bathtub, are thought to be safe.

7. Has your child any pain or redness along the sides of the nails?

Children are agile. You might consider it a feat to bite your toenails, but Junior probably can—

and possibly does. Second in "agility-fun" to biting is tearing toenails. And with a real thriller on television, what better emotional outlet?

Biting and tearing will sometimes cause pain or infection because spicules of nail are left in the nail grooves to impinge on the soft tissue. There may even be a tear directly into the surrounding flesh. If it has come to such a pass, make an appointment with your podiatrist. In the meantime, have Junior soak his foot for ten minutes at a time in comfortably warm, *not hot,* water. Use just plain warm water, no salts or fancy medication in the water. The warmth of the water is all you need.

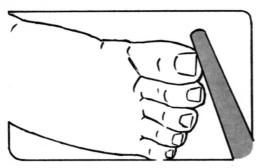

To try to avoid the temptation of such indulgences as nail biting or tearing, keep your child's nails cut straight across, just about to the tip of the toe. Don't cut into the corners of a normal nail. Use an emery board after cutting to eliminate a spur onto which Junior can latch.

There is one complaint for which you need not be alert, because the cries of pain—often in the middle of the night—will bring you on the run. These are the severe pains of leg cramping experienced by many children, often between the ages of two and five. There are various explanations for these cramps, which we no longer accept simply as growing pains. Some of the explanations are faulty gait, lowering of the temperature of the bedroom, one leg resting on the other during sleep. Fatigue, however, is probably the most valid explanation. Such fatigue may be caused by the activity of the day or by poor foot posture with a secondary deficiency in over-all body posture.

Generally, massaging the foot and leg will alleviate the immediate pain. It is also advisable to maintain an even temperature in the bedroom during the night, perhaps with a safe electric heater operating on a thermostat. Of course, if there is a recurrence of such cramping, your pediatrician should be consulted.

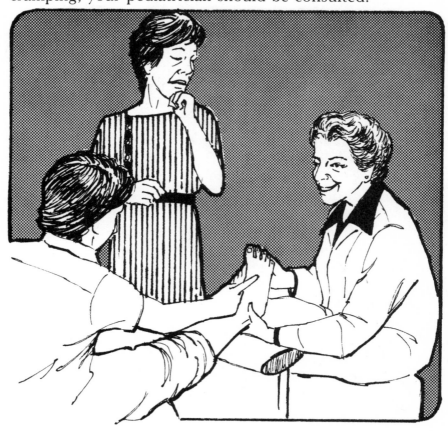

As a doctor, I make one plea to you. When you and Junior are in the doctor's office, let Junior do the talking. Give the doctor and the patient a chance to establish a good relationship. Don't treat Junior like a commodity. He may need help in describing his reason for being there, but don't proffer help unless it is absolutely necessary. As a parent, I know the overwhelming self-restraint this demands. You may be surprised, though, to find that Junior will tell the doctor some things he hasn't told you!

Walking barefoot on soft surfaces, such as the unpaved ground, sand and rugs, is great and, except for the usual assortment of cuts and injuries that may result, is desirable. Most children, however, must wear shoes for the greater part of the day. And here is another point of alertness required of you. In the selection of shoes for your child you really have no guidance beyond your own alertness and the advice of your podiatrist. It is a rare shoe salesman who is a shoe fitter, though he may have been given a special title in the shoe store or in the children's shoe section of a department store and may be assigned to check the shoe fittings of other clerks.

Some years ago I took my daughter to a New York department store, well known for its children's shoes. We were approached by a pleasant, intelligent young man. I disagreed, however, with his opinion of the fit of each of the pairs of shoes he tried on Jude. Finally I asked him for a larger size in one of the styles he had shown us. When he put it on her, he promptly declared it too big. I just as promptly said, "That fits Jude. We'll take it."

The salesman, realizing that I was knowledgeable about shoes, asked why I thought that shoe was correct. This led to a lengthy discussion during which he admitted that, although his was a title of chief shoe fitter, and every child's fit had to be approved by him, he really knew nothing about fitting shoes. He had been given his title and assignment because he had passed a written test with a higher grade than that of any of the other salespeople in the department!

Shoes for children should be fitted so that, *when standing,* each shoe is approximately one-half inch longer than the longest toe (which is not necessarily the big toe). They should be deep enough from top to bottom not to press down on the toes. The heel fit should be snug. You 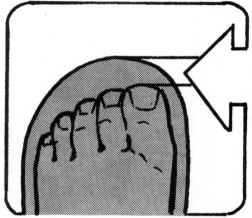 should be able to ripple the leather or fabric of the shoe across the top of the foot with your finger. Shoes should approximate the shape of the foot.

In my opinion, shoes for children should be flexible. Heavy, rigid shoes, certainly for a young child, simply make walking more difficult. This is particularly true for the child who has any neurologic or over-all muscular problem.

When children first start walking, high shoes are often suggested. Don't for one moment believe the salesman who tells you that they will support the ankles. The only advantage of a high shoe for a very young child is that it is easier to keep on and harder for him to take off himself. Support of the ankles

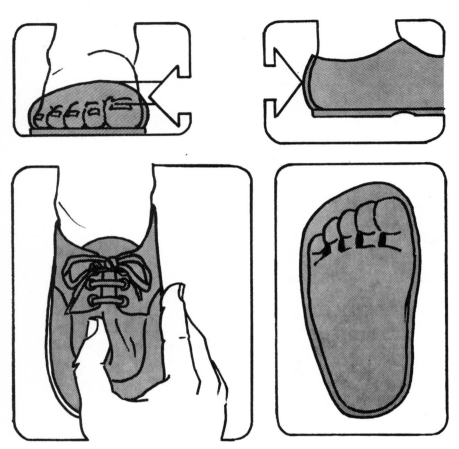

comes from correct positioning of the feet, not from binding the ankles.

With school comes the beginning of the peer-conscious period. "Joe has loafers. Why can't I?"

Remembering that we're interested in a total person, not just in the feet, there follows some soul searching, based on all the traditions of the superiority of an oxford and counter-balanced by the psychiatric warnings of dire things for your child if you interfere with peer conformity. The life of a parent is many-faceted, indeed!

For the normal foot a loafer that *fits properly* is quite acceptable. For the less-than-normal foot, your podiatrist's decision must hold sway.

Sneakers, particularly because of their flexibility, are fine. For the older girl, for whom sneakers are generally tapered, it is wisest to buy boys' sneakers, which always have rounded toes. In our unisex world of today, this represents no style tug-of-war.

Sandals are good as long as the straps or openings do not cause pressure on any part of the foot.

Mary Janes for dress-up occasions are an essential part of most little girls' wardrobes. First start out with the understanding that they are dress-up, not everyday. Then be sure they are properly fitted. Most of them are of patent leather which is not porous and has no give, making them undesirable for full time use.

From season to season other styles appear, first in adult shoes, and then in children's sizes, with the consumer's dollar rather than his foot requirements the chief incentive for copying the adult styles. Some of them are deplorable, such as the heavy weight, snug boots for boys. Some of them are not bad, even if not good, such as the boys' buckle shoes.

This concept of copying adult shoe styles, in much the same manner that toy manufacturers produce small stoves and brooms and automobiles, often leaves the older child, particularly a girl of perhaps ten to twelve, in a hiatus period—where little girl shoes may fit the foot but not the eye, and the more sophisticated, often higher heeled, shoe may fit the eye but not the foot.

There are two firm admonitions about children's shoes, admonitions to be stressed the more because the expense of shoes for two or three or four children can be great.

1. No hand-me-downs.

   Each youngster wears shoes differently from any other child. It is a gross injustice to give the next younger child shoes already adapted to all the peculiarities of another's feet.

2. No resoling of children's shoes.

   Children's feet grow too quickly to permit shoe repairs other than new tips and heel lifts. Their shoes should never be resoled. As a matter of fact, I don't think anybody's shoes should be resoled since the shoe almost always becomes smaller in the process of resoling.

Drying wet shoes near heat will cause shrinkage. When Junior comes home rain- or snow-soaked, stuff his shoes with crumpled tissue paper or newspaper and put them off in a corner well away from the heat. Thorough drying may take two or three days.

In his book *Walk and Be Happy,* Dr. Benjamin Kauth, a prominent New York podiatrist, suggests the following schedule to approximate the time intervals for new shoes.

Age	Size changes every:
1 to 6 years	4 to 8 weeks
6 to 10 years	8 to 12 weeks
10 to 12 years	12 to 16 weeks
12 to 15 years	16 to 20 weeks
15 years and over	6 months and up

This schedule is a reflection of the growth of the foot at various ages, not of the time it takes to wear out a shoe. It is economical in both money and health to discard shoes that are no longer large enough, even though they are still in good condition.

For some time it has been illegal in New York to fit shoes by "x-ray." It had been the delight of children buying new shoes to stand on a box that gave a fluoroscopic picture of the feet in the shoes. It was determined that these children, with repeated exposure, were being exposed to an excessive amount of x-ray. If these devices are still in use in your area, I would advise against allowing your child to be fitted this way.

After your child has worn new shoes for a day, check his feet for any irritated spots. Frequently shoes that are too stiff will irritate the back of a youngster's heel. You can sometimes overcome this by "rolling" the back of the shoe. Grasp the back of 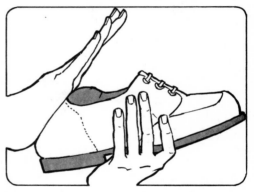 the shoe with the heel of your hand and gently bend it inward to soften it.

There is no such thing as a "corrective" shoe, either for a child or for an adult. Shoes at best are foot coverings. At worst they are irritants and cripplers. If you suspect a need for any "correction," take Junior to your podiatrist.

If he does need professional care to maintain his feet in the correct position, then your podiatrist will suggest any one of several ways of doing this. He may suggest a support in the shoe or a separate support or wedging. Beware, though, of the doctor who makes so light of this that he sends you to a laboratory for some appliance that he never checks or to a shoe store for shoes with corrections that he never sees.

Hosiery that is too small can be extremely harmful to your youngster's feet. In the early years the hosiery should be rounded at the toes, as close to the shape of the foot as possible. At all times you must guard against shrinkage or the wearing of socks, stockings, tights or pantyhose beyond the growth period of adequate fit.

The Podiatry Society of the State of New York has compiled the following table of children's shoe and hosiery sizes, which certainly should not be followed rigidly, but which does offer valid guidance.

Age	Shoe	Hose
3 months	0	4
6 months	1	4½
1–1½	2–3	5
2–2½	4–5	5½
3–4	6–7	6
4–5	8–9	6½
6–7	10–11	7
8–9	12–13	7½
10–11	1–2	8
12–13	2–3	8½
13–14	3½–4½	9

Woolen socks or heavy cotton socks offer a youngster's feet some protection and buffer for sports. Use woolen socks for winter wear. Sometimes a woolen sock over a cotton sock is desirable. If Junior uses both, be sure both are large enough for his feet and not too bulky for his shoes or boots.

I would be remiss, indeed, were I not to anticipate

your questions about Caroline who, with hopes of being the prima ballerina, wants to start right now. Perhaps the urgency is the greater because every little girl in the neighborhood is going to be a prima ballerina and how can you deprive your daughter of her future?

Ballet lessons—or any dancing lessons—can be good exercise with stress on optimum coordination. Ballet, of course, calls for shoes that are more snug than most other types, but these will do little damage during the relatively brief periods of instruction. New ballet shoes, however, should be bought when the growth of the foot indicates a new shoe wardrobe.

A ballet teacher should be selected with care. A knowledgeable, responsible teacher will not permit even a gifted student to do toe work before enough groundwork has been covered and until the muscles and bones are sufficiently developed so that no physical deformity will result. This is generally no

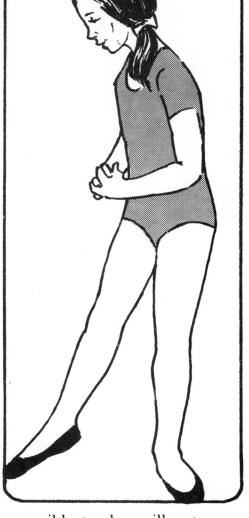

59

earlier than the age of ten and it may be later. If in your community there is an organization of dancing instructors, you might inquire about a reputable teacher.

Celia Sparger, physiotherapist of the Sadler Wells School, has written an excellent brochure entitled, *Why Can't I Go on My Toes?* It is available from Capezio, 543 West 43rd Street, New York, New York 10063.

Sparger highlights the fact that, ". . . It is easier to say when a child should not begin *pointe* work than to give a definite age limit or lay down the length of training to precede it." She also cites the possibility of lifelong deformity consequent upon *pointe* work before the muscles and bones are sufficiently developed.

Correct *pointe* work demands that the foot be on the tips of the four smaller toes and on the pad of the big toe. Proper ballet shoe construction is essential to implement this. Capezio also publishes two interesting pamphlets demonstrating the desirable construction and proper lacing of ballet shoes. These are *The Care and Fit of Toe Shoes* and *Tools of the Dance*.

From the point of view of community action, I urge you to request and to encourage school surveys of foot health. The Podiatry Society of the State of New York has been particularly helpful to parents not only in distributing gratis literature on the care of children's feet, but also in conducting school surveys, at the conclusion of which a report on each child's foot health is sent home with recommendations for the treatment of abnormalities. If such school surveys have not been held in your area, contact the local podiatry society, requesting a foot survey for your child's school.

60

Chapter 6

No Matter How Much They Hurt, Corns and Callus Are NOT Your Problem

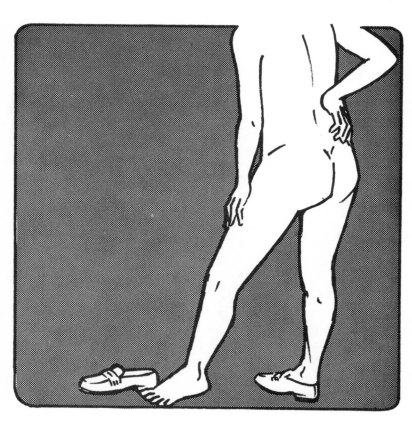

Your corns and callus may hurt you so much that you limp, but *they* are NOT your problem.

Your corns and callus may be your reason for making an appointment to see your podiatrist, but they are NOT your problem.

They are only symptoms of your problem, just as a cough is only a symptom of a respiratory disturbance. You may want your doctor to give you medication to minimize the discomfort and fatigue resulting from the strain of coughing, but I'll wager you'll not be content unless you know he is also treating you for the underlying respiratory condition. Actually, you should be grateful that there is a symptom, no matter how discomforting in itself, to warn of the basic condition.

So, too, with corns and callus. Think of them as signals of some other pathology.

Under a microscope corns and callus are identical cellular structures. There is an increase of epidermal cells, causing pressure on the papillae of the skin.

The callus, however, develops in flat planes, while

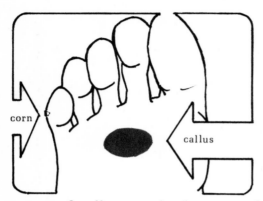

corn

callus

the corn is shaped like a cone with the tip penetrating into the tissue. This is why a corn is so painful on direct pressure. An example too many of us know well is the pressure of a snug shoe against a corn on the fifth toe. If one area of callus on the bottom of the foot becomes intolerably painful, there may even be a corn with a callus.

You must remember that any acutely painful area within a callus requires the immediate attention of your podiatrist since it might be any one of several other lesions, such as an ulcer, a pseudo-sinus, a hematoma or a wart. These, too, are essentially symptomatic of some underlying condition, unless you have had an injury to your foot.

Corns and callus are formed by prolonged recurrent friction and pressure. The friction and pressure, by irritation, increase the blood supply to the area, causing an acceleration of cell growth. The additional cells form the corn or callus.

Recurrent pressure and friction on a small site, such as a toe, will result in a corn. Recurrent pressure and friction on a larger area, such as the ball of the foot, will result in callus. It is the combination of both types of pressure and friction that gives rise to a corn within a callus. This sometimes occurs on the ball of the foot, when, within the larger area, there is a small bony prominence that is receiving the brunt of concentrated pressure and friction.

Soft corns are always found between toes, frequently in pairs, one facing the other. The immediate causative factor is the rubbing of one toe against the other at a site of bony prominences.

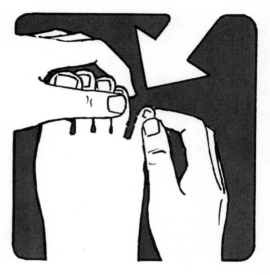

Seed corns generally develop in groups. They are small, sometimes only pinhead in size. They are most often found on the sole of the foot, frequently the result of a series of small irritants such as lasting tacks in a shoe.

It is not only on the foot that corns and callus appear. You are undoubtedly familiar with the callus that so often develops on the inner side of the third finger of the person who constantly uses a pen or pencil. Always, though, a corn or callus is the result of abnormal pressure and friction. Just because you have corns or callus or both, don't assume that everybody

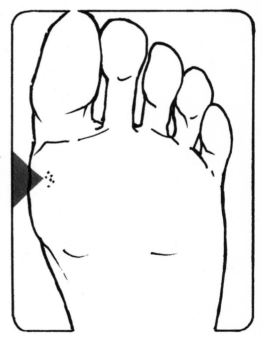

65

else has. Many are the feet I have seen with no trace of corns or callus, and I say this in spite of the fact that almost all the patients I see have some foot complaint.

Now that we know what a corn and a callus are and that they come from recurrent pressure and friction, what causes them?

If your answer is poorly fitting shoes, you're wrong! Think of all the people you know who wear wide, conservative, unattractive shoes—and still have corns and callus. Think of all the people you know who wear ridiculously high styled, ill fitting shoes and never complain about their feet.

No, it's not simply the shoes, but primarily your feet that are the problem.

Where are your feet in your shoes when once you start walking? Do they slip all the way to the front so that any shoe becomes too small for you regardless of how big it might be in relationship to your resting foot?

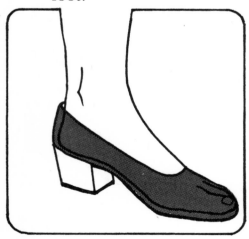

YOUR FOOT DOES NOT GROW AFTER YOU ARE 18 TO 20 YEARS OLD. Yet the chances are that you've taken larger and larger shoes since you were twenty, only to find that soon each new size seemed too small. Obviously, if your foot is constantly sliding all the way forward, as far as your shoes will permit, then the shoes are too small, though they may be gapping at the heel. This is true for both men and women, though the traditionally higher heel on a woman's shoe aggravates the process. This is one reason most women agree that open-toe shoes are more comfortable than closed-toe shoes; as their feet slide forward there is no toe box against which their toes hit.

Put your hand, palm up, along the upper part of the inside of the front of one of your older closed-toe shoes. It is very likely that you will find an indentation, possibly even a hole, made by your great toe as it has constantly slipped forward, resulting in pressure from both the top and the very front of the shoe. This indentation is probably not at the inner side of the shoe where the great toe

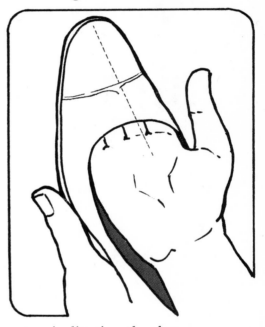

should be, but well to the center, indicating the degree to which the position of your foot is distorted within the shoe. In part, this is the result of the tapering of the shoe, but, in greater part, the result of the elongation of your foot because the muscles and bones of the foot and leg are not functioning in the right relationship to each other.

Look at the bottom of your shoe. Are you wearing out the outer part of the heel, but the inner part of the sole? Or, even if the outer side of the sole does show any wear, is the greater wear on the inner part

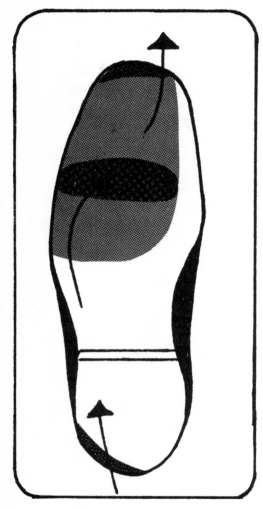

of the sole? In a shoe with extreme tapering, women in particular may find tread marks only on a small middle section of the sole, indicating that the foot is so compressed in the shoe that there can be only a minimal weight bearing area. Does the inner part of the upper of the shoe bulge away from the foot?

Ideally the shoe becomes worn at the heel and along the outer border of the sole because the foot is making contact with the ground first at the heel, then along the outer border and finally across the ball of the foot to the great toe. To the degree that this is not so, the foot tends to point away from the body, Charlie Chaplin fashion, instead of pointing fairly straight ahead. At the same time the foot rolls over toward the midline of the body causing a bulge in the inner border of the upper of the shoe. This is the typical picture of pronation, so common in both men and women.

Now we have an understanding of the foot slipping

forward, rolling to the inner side and pointing away from the body, with the abnormal function of the foot causing recurrent pressure and friction resulting in corns and callus. This is perhaps the most frequent cause of corns and callus.

The effects are more far-reaching, however. Many a patient complaining of corns and callus readily admits to increased fatigue, lower back pain, and cramping of the feet and/or legs. Such cramping often occurs during the night, forcing the patient to pop out of bed in acute pain. Sometimes, too, there are complaints of knee pain or of leg pain when walking.

It has always interested me that the majority of patients who have consulted me because of corns and callus are surprised when I ask questions about these other symptoms. They have never thought of the corns and callus in connection with their other problems. Some of them have had treatment which was unsuccessful. Leg pains, for instance, have been treated with oral medication, but this did not take into account the various related symptoms.

I have no desire to oversimplify this whole matter, nor is my goal to have you become a self-diagnostician. I shall not attempt to detail for you all the points of differential diagnosis involving back problems, which may have any of several origins or a combination of origins. Some of these back problems are not caused by faulty foot posture at all. Some, however, do aggravate the foot condition, and are, in turn, aggravated by the foot condition.

I shall not attempt to detail for you all the possible causes of fatigue, but I sure can shout loudly that you can't have your feet out of line without affecting the rest of your body. And you don't have corns or callus unless you have at least the potential for other symptoms!

Nor can you rule out the possibilities of ailments of the rest of your body affecting your feet. Callus may come from a difference in the length of your legs or from arthritic changes. Your great toe may be painful —or numb—because of shoe pressure against the toe as you slide forward in your shoe, rolling over on the great toe, forming callus along the border of the toe. Your great toe may be painful because the faulty position of the foot in the shoe has caused a corn to form in the nail groove. Your great toe may be painful because of a bunion or because of arthritis. Your great toe may be numb because of an impingement on a nerve resulting from a disc problem in the vertebral column or because of a growth on the spinal cord.

It's easy to see why I urge you against self-diagnosis as strongly as I urge you to consult your podiatrist for any foot problem—including your corns and callus.

It is true, in justice to your corn, that it can serve as a barometer. With an increase of moisture in the air, there is a compensating increase in the tissue fluid in the area, aggravating the irritability of the nerve endings. But isn't it easier and more comfortable to get a weather report on the radio or television?

Don't use over-the-counter "corn cures." They don't cure. They generally contain an acid which destroys the surrounding healthy tissue and often causes an ulceration at the site of the corn. Healing the ulceration may be a lengthy, painful and expensive matter.

Incidentally, a corn has no root, although some "corn cures" claim to "remove the root." There may be a deeper portion at the site of the greatest degree of friction and pressure, but there is no root. Corns on your feet and flourishing Flora just don't have the same origin!

Don't use a pumice stone or a metal file on your callus. All you succeed in doing is to irritate the area.

If your corn is so pain-
ful that you want to pro-
tect it until you have
proper treatment, don't
buy a corn pad with an
oval opening or with an
oval depression which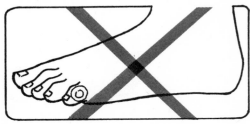
frequently contains an acid preparation. (Remember that the acid is dangerous for tissue.) The oval will cause pressure on the surrounding area, making the corn or callus bulge into the opening.

If you've already
bought a pad with an
oval or round opening,
cut out a wedge, making
it horseshoe shaped.
Place the pad sufficiently
far behind the corn so
that, as you go forward
in your shoe, it won't rub
against the corn it is supposed to protect. If the
pad is impregnated with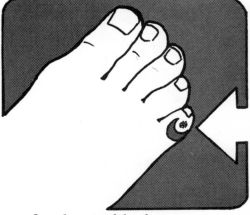
any medication, the best area for that pad is the gar-
bage pail. Don't use medicated pads!

A much better type of pad to protect a corn is a "spot" type band-aid, which also has the advantage of a sterile gauze center. Put the sterile gauze directly over the corn. Avoid the rectangular type of band-aid that must be wrapped completely around the toe. The

71

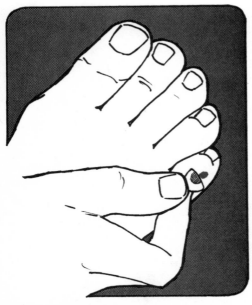

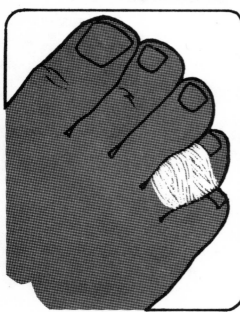

bulk may cause irritation and the constriction may be too great for comfort.

Soft corns are best protected by strands of a good quality lamb's wool. Don't use the coarse type found in beauty parlors. The strands should be drawn out into a thin, even layer and then wrapped *loosely* around the toe. If two adjacent toes are involved, only one need be wrapped with the lamb's wool. Be sure to remove the wool before bathing.

The best protection for callus is a thin piece of moleskin placed directly over the callus, but separated from it by gauze or absorbent cotton. In removing the moleskin each day be *sure* to hold the skin of the sole of your foot taut while you SLOWLY pull the moleskin BACK TOWARDS THE HEEL. Forget all you've ever heard about removing adhesives quickly. Do it

SLOWLY and GO BACK TOWARDS THE HEEL. If you don't, you may find a wide, bleeding gash where you've ripped the flesh along with the moleskin.

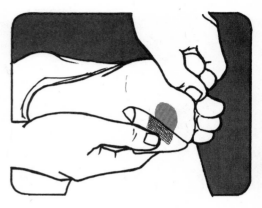

It is advisable to leave both corn and callus coverings off during the night, as well as when you're bathing. This avoids an excessive accumulation of moisture and helps to maintain the healthy tone of the surrounding tissue. (Of course, if your doctor has put a dressing on your corn or callus, it's his decision as to whether or not it is to be removed.)

Don't under any circumstances indulge in "bathroom surgery," during which, with razor grasped in one hand, you hold your breath as rigidly as you hold your foot with your other hand. Maybe, to date, you haven't had a blood-bath accident in your self-surgery, but there's always a tomorrow!

And remember that as long as you limit your office visits to your corner drugstore or to your own bathroom, you'll never learn what your corns and callus really do signify.

Chapter 7

Is It Really an Ingrown Toenail?

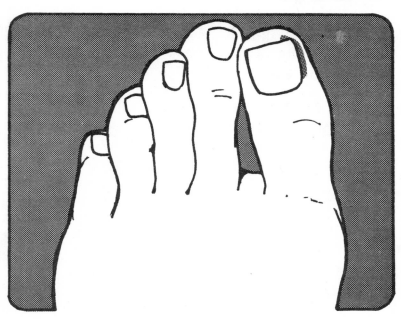

Ingrown nails don't grow in.

What really happens is that the flesh around the nail is forced so close against the sides of the nail that the nail seems to be growing into the flesh.

The advice for home treatment of an ingrown toenail used to be to cut a wedge out of the top edge of the nail. The theory was that the nail would grow to the center, relieving the pressure at the sides. Hopefully this theory has been put to rest along with many other medical myths.

A nail grows straight forward from an area called the matrix. The matrix is behind the point where the nail is seen emerging from the toe. The nail attaches to the nail bed as it grows forward from the matrix. The nail bed appears 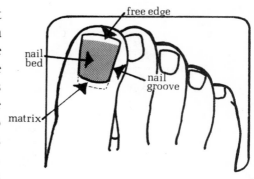 normally as the pink area showing through the larger portion of the nail. The white part of the nail, the part

75

you cut, is the free end that has grown beyond the nail bed.

Cutting a wedge in the nail will not affect growth since the nail grows forward from the matrix. It takes about 120 days for a normal nail to develop from the matrix to the end of the toe. If the nail is abnormal, no one can predict the rate of growth.

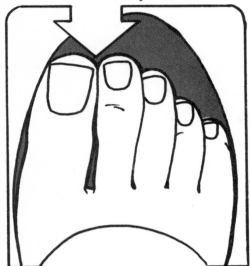

Ingrown nails most often appear on the great toe, but they are sometimes found on the smaller toes. They may be caused by the consistent use of pointed shoes that periodically are considered stylish for both men and women. Short, tight hosiery can also cause ingrown nails. This is particularly true of "support" hosiery that constricts the toes.

Even in properly fitting shoes and hosiery ingrown nails may develop from pressure if the foot rolls to the inner side and pushes forward. The toes are crushed together, pushing the flesh at the sides tight against the nail. This occurs often on the great toe, where the shoe presses against one side of the nail and the second toe presses against the other side. Callus may form in the nail groove from the pressure and friction of the nail against the flesh. If there is an area of particularly concentrated pressure and friction, a corn may develop in the groove—and it can be mighty painful!

76

If, however, the flesh is actually penetrated by the side of the nail, the chances are great that an infection will occur. Not only will the area be red and hot and painful, but your podiatrist may find a large amount of pus in the nail groove.

The only home treatment you should attempt for a *noninfected* ingrown nail is simply to work a few strands of absorbent cotton between the nail and the flesh. Draw out the strands of cotton in a thin layer before inserting the packing. Use the blunt end of an orange stick from a manicuring kit to insert it.

If you suspect infection, soak your foot in plain warm water, NOT HOT WATER, for ten minutes at a time at least three times a day—until you get to the earliest appointment your podiatrist can give you. When you go to your podiatrist's office, take along an old shoe you won't fret about should the doctor want to cut it to relieve pressure. The less pressure you have on the infected area, the more rapid the healing.

ANY SHOE OR SLIP-PER CAUSES SOME PRESSURE unless, in the case of women, it is a mule or open-toe shoe the top of which ends well behind the toes. A thong sandal, such as a beach sandal, will also avoid pressure.

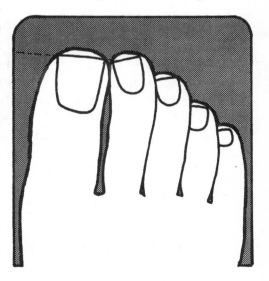

Many people cause their own nail problems by cutting the nails im-properly. You should cut your nails straight across

77

the top without going into the nail grooves. Your podiatrist may cut the sides of the nail at the nail grooves, but he knows how and when to do it. He, moreover, has the sterile instruments and is at the right end of your foot. You're much further away from your foot, no matter how agile you are!

For some ingrown nails your podiatrist may decide surgery is necessary to remove part of the matrix and the overlapping flesh. For others he may prefer simply cutting away part of the nail, leaving the matrix intact,

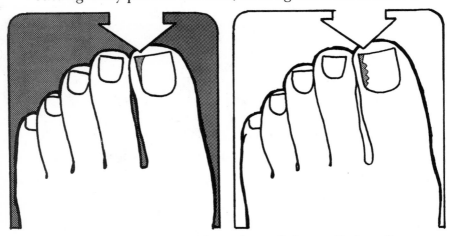

but smoothly curving the edge of the nail that faces the nail groove. Almost always when a patient attempts to go down into the nail groove to cut away part of the nail, there are left spicules of nail, shaped like fish hooks, that cut into the flesh. The toe may be so irritated that all these spicules cannot be removed at one visit. The irritation may cause a mass of painful tissue to form at the edge of the nail groove. This is called proud flesh. You may have heard it referred to as *wilde Fleisch.*

78

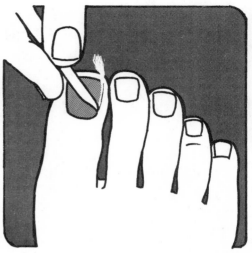

DON'T ATTEMPT TO CUT AWAY THE SIDE OF THE NAIL, WHETHER OR NOT YOU ARE HAVING PAIN. Inserting a wisp of cotton is a far safer procedure!

Many other abnormalities occur in nails, some of them painless for a long time. Pain, of course, is a wonderful thing. We may not enjoy it, but it is a warning without which an abnormal condition progresses sometimes to the point of danger. For this reason I urge you to consult your podiatrist if any of your nails begins to look different from the others.

Many nail problems, like so many problems in other parts of the body, develop insidiously, without being noticed until they are so advanced that not only is there pain, but the time and expense for treatment become many times greater than would have been necessary had professional care been sought earlier.

A common nail problem is a fungous growth (athlete's foot) under the nail. The nail frequently develops dirty-looking yellow streaks or, if neglected, becomes entirely discolored. This should not be confused with the white streaks that are often the result of injury to the nail and that usually disappear as the nail grows forward.

Neglected fungous conditions of the nails may cause

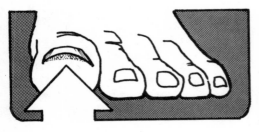 an extremely unpleasant odor. A mass of powdery debris develops under the nail, sometimes elevating the center and causing the sides to dip down into the flesh. Unless the sides actually impinge on the flesh there is no pain—no danger signal except the appearance of the nail. A fungous condition of the nail is known as *onychomycosis*. It frequently coexists with a fungous condition between the toes or on the soles of the feet, and can be a source of infection for other parts of the body.

Today treatment of *onychomycosis* is lengthy, but several years ago there was no known way of treating it!

Don't make your own diagnosis of athlete's foot of the nail and then hurry down to the local drugstore to buy one of a raft of over-the-counter cures for athlete's foot. In the first place, most medications for athlete's foot, even if they are effective on the skin, will be totally ineffective on the nail.

Secondly, you have to be a very experienced clinician to differentiate between *onychomycosis* and other nail conditions. Even your doctor will probably want to take a specimen of shavings from the nail and of the debris under it to grow a culture for verification of the diagnosis.

Psoriasis of the nail is readily confused by the layman with a fungous infection.

The toes are subject to frequent injuries, often with disfiguring of the nails. Such injuries may be massive and easily explained. One example would be having a gallon jug of wine fall on your foot.

There may be, however, a series of small injuries,

whose origin is less apparent to you. This happens if your great toenail constantly hits against the top and front of your shoe. If there is a small injury with each step, you eventually have the equivalent of a massive injury.

As a consequence of injury, the nail may become thickened, the growth taking place more in thickness than in length. The center portion of the nail becomes particularly thick and the sides tend to invert into the flesh of the nail grooves. This is popu- 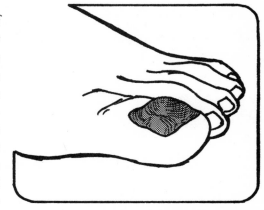 larly called a club nail. Pressure of the shoe down on the thickened nail causes pain. Additionally, the inverted sides of the nail irritate the surrounding flesh.

All injuries to nails do not cause this type of disfiguring. An injury may cause a *hematoma* under the nail. This is a blood clot that becomes painful because of the pressure of the nail. Having the overlying part of the nail removed and the blood clot drained is less painful than you might think. Treatment is essential not simply to eliminate pain, but to avoid permanent injury to the nail bed. The nail, which grows out straight from the matrix, cannot grow normally if the nail bed, to which it attaches, is not normal—just as a train cannot run smoothly over a bumpy track. A nail with a bump in it has probably had to grow over a bumpy nail bed.

As a hobby some people paint pictures, some play pinochle, some sail boats. And some tear their nails

81

—often paying the price of pain and infection. I've tried having patients coat the ends of their toes, including the nails, with colorless nail polish. I've seldom been successful. Television watching hasn't helped. It's such a great time for nail tearing. And psychotherapy is expensive! If this is your hobby, why not try push-ups instead?

If you're diabetic, NEVER CUT YOUR OWN NAILS. Even though your nails may seem to be things of beauty, DO NOT CUT THEM YOURSELF. See your podiatrist regularly on a monthly basis and NEVER CUT YOUR OWN NAILS.

Women sometimes ask whether there is any objection to painting their toenails. Unless you have an allergy to the nail polish, there is no objection. Do, however, avoid globs of polish in the nail grooves where it hardens and can irritate the flesh. And, please, please, remove nail polish before you visit your podiatrist. It's impossible for him to check abnormalities on nails that are coated with polish!

A popular addition to the beauty salon routine is the pedicure. An unskilled operator may go beyond the safe or legal limits of care. Nail groove work should be avoided. Cuticles should not be cut, but gently rolled back. Polish should be kept out of the grooves.

One last caution about nails I have kept for the end of this chapter—for sheer emphasis. I have discussed the reasons for some changes in the appearance of the nails, with the advice to consult your podiatrist. An additional reason for consulting him, however, is that the changes may be a manifestation of systemic disease and may lead him to seek consultation with your internist or general practitioner.

Chapter **8**

Warts, Rashes and
Perspiring Feet

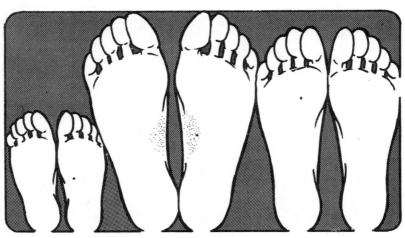

If there is a wart on YOUR foot, examine the feet of everyone in your household for any growth even remotely resembling yours! Warts are contagious.

Warts are said to appear chiefly on the feet of children and teenagers, but they are found on the feet of people of all ages, including the elderly.

A wart is known medically as a *verruca.* It is a benign tumor. You're probably familiar with warts on the hands and on other non-weight-bearing surfaces. They have a small cauliflower texture protruding above the skin, sometimes by a thin necklike attachment. Warts on the foot most frequently appear on the sole, particularly at sites of abnormal weight bearing. The constant irritation of these areas may provide a portal of entry for the filterable virus that causes the wart. This is the reason that treatment for such warts involves not only surgery or chemotherapy, but also padding to eliminate the weight bearing from that area. It is the reason, too, that, after the wart has been cured, the patient is often advised to have treatment to correct faulty weight bearing.

A wart on the sole is called a plantar *verruca,* be-

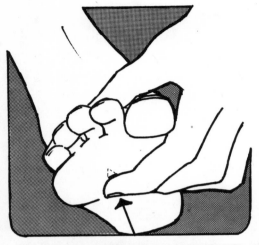

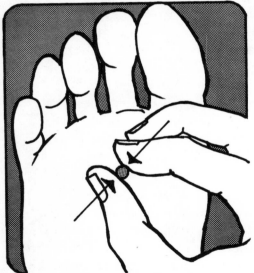

cause, as I mentioned before, the bottom surface of the foot is the plantar surface. As a result of weight bearing the wart is forced into the foot. On the surface it resembles a corn. It is often covered by callus. Although a wart may appear to be a corn, different characteristics become apparent on closer examination.

A corn is painful when pressure is applied directly on it.

A wart is painful when pressure is applied on both sides of it.

A corn does not have blood vessels.

A wart has many blood vessels. You may see dark dots within a wart. They are capillary endings.

Warts on the bottom of the foot may become very painful. We speak of the mother wart and of satellites because first one growth appears. Then others, many others, may develop, even on the other foot.

Not only do they spread, but they are contagious. If one member of the family has warts, the chances are

86

others will develop them. This is particularly true of those who share a bathmat or other wet porous materials like towels. For cleanliness and safety, each person in a family should have his own bathmat and his own towel, just as he has his own toothbrush. Other conditions, like athlete's foot, can be carried from one person to another by wet porous materials. A bathtub, the porcelain of which is non-porous, is thought to be safe.

Autumn or early winter is when the greatest number of patients with warts on their feet present themselves at podiatrists' offices. This is probably because they have been infected during the summer by walking barefoot on the wet, porous floors of shower-rooms and bathhouses. Shower rooms in schools are frequently suspect. Water seems to accelerate the growth of warts. Consequently the doctor usually instructs the patient to keep his foot dry during the period of treatment.

For a special occasion—such as a long-awaited vacation—that may occur during treatment, there is one trick that works well, if the warts are not too numerous. The patient covers the growths with colorless nail polish, leaving a wide border of polish around the area. This permits him to go swimming without getting the warts wet. It is not ideal

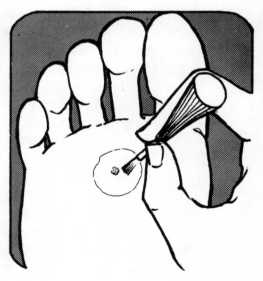

for routine care because it eliminates the advantage of a protective padding.

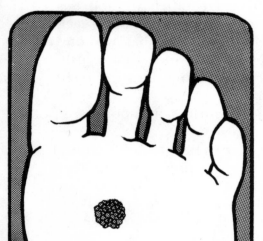

Various kinds of warts are found on the foot. Some are single lesions. Some are clusters of lesions that seem to form a mosaic pattern. These mosaic warts are difficult to cure, but given enough time for treatment (sometimes many months), they can be eliminated.

Warts hold a special interest for the dermatologist and the podiatrist because their response to treatment is not always predictable. Some people seem particularly susceptible to these growths. I've seen patients with warts covering half of the sole of each foot. I've cleared up the warts, accurately charting on my records where they had appeared, only to have the patient call a few months later to say he had more warts. Checking against the records proved they were new growths, not a recurrence of the original ones.

Warts in certain people seem to be psychogenic. They appear when the patient is under emotional stress and recede during the periods of greater emotional stability. *This does not contradict the fact that warts are generally caused by a virus and do require treatment.*

I recall a boy of fourteen who always arrived at the office accompanied by his high-strung mother and frequently by his more high-strung maternal grandmother. Jerry had so many warts on each foot that I finally stopped counting. His hands were similarly covered. The initial growth had appeared on his foot. When this is so, the warts on the hands will often disappear when those on the feet are cured.

Jerry was conscientious in coming the day of each of his appointments. He and his distaff entourage, however, always were late and always arrived in a dither. While the ladies bewailed Jerry's fate, Jerry fretted about two things. One was the fact that from visit to visit new warts appeared on his hands and feet. The other was his mother's problems. Sometimes she had a headache. Sometimes she had a bellyache. Another time her girdle was uncomfortable for her.

That girdle was my clue. In one fell swoop I killed two birds with one shot! I gave Jerry the name of a corsetiere and I told him that, what with continuing treatment, his warts would begin to disappear almost overnight. I instructed him to draw an outline of each hand and of each foot, to put in a dot for each wart and then to cross out the dot as the wart disappeared.

Seven days later Momma had a new girdle and about one third of his dots had been crossed out. The girdle fit well. It had been an expensive indulgence. Momma was happy. Grandma had gone to visit another offspring. No new dots appeared and crosses within the outlines multiplied. His feet were beginning to look great. I was real proud of myself.

Then Grandma returned. Momma developed flu. New warts zoomed into view.

We repeated this flux and recession for a few months. Suggesting a psychiatrist instead of a podiatrist would have been an outrage in the opinion of these people.

Finally Jerry disappeared from my scene when Momma and Grandma both developed bad colds. I can only hope that, as Jerry reached chronologic manhood, he managed his emotional divorce. If so, perhaps his warts have disappeared.

I have cited an extreme case. I have seen others, less dramatic than this, some in people much older than Jerry. I am never content, however, to start off on the premise that the warts are psychogenic. *Warts should be treated.*

The skin on the sole of the foot is thicker than that on any other part of the body. It is covered with ridges that make the footprint as individual as the fingerprint. It contains more sweat glands and pressure sensitive nerve endings than any other part of the body.

Various skin problems, other than warts, occur on the sole of the foot. This is due partly to the nature of the skin on the sole of the foot and partly to weight bearing with the consequent irritation from shoes or from rough surfaces when walking barefoot.

Blisters, if they must be treated at home, should *not* be opened by a needle that has been flamed. The area should first be cleaned thoroughly with an antiseptic. Rubbing alcohol is in most home medicine cabinets. It is an excellent antiseptic. A new needle should be cleaned in the alcohol. The blister can then be punctured with reasonable safety and the fluid gently pressed from the blister. After this the site should be washed again with alcohol, even though it stings. It's a good sting! The area should be covered with a sterile band-aid or a piece of sterile gauze.

Breaks in the skin between the toes or around the heels sometimes occur. They are called *fissures* and can be extremely painful. Fissures between the toes usually develop because of inadequate drying after bathing or because of drying too roughly. Putting your foot up on the washbasin or on the side of the tub to dry thoroughly, but gently, is great exercise. Try it! Your skin will be healthier and you'll be more agile.

If the fissures are deep, it may be necessary to use a medication. Compound tincture of benzoin can be bought without a prescription. If it is painted on the fissured areas twice a day, it forms a protective film that is not washed off by water. After two or three days it can be removed with rubbing alcohol. This process of building up a film and then removing it when it becomes uncomfortably thick can be repeated until the fissures are healed. (Any medication that has the word "tincture" in its name is soluble in alcohol, rather than water.)

The compound tincture of benzoin may be dispensed in a bottle labeled with instructions to use the contents with steam as an inhalant for a respiratory condition. You can inhale from now until doomsday, but it won't help the fissures! Use it directly on the fissures.

Certain foot powders help to keep the toe areas dry after the fissures have healed. Because talcum powder cakes, I don't advise using it. Cornstarch is helpful.

Again, however, I warn you about self-diagnosis. You must be sure that your fissures are fissures, not some other condition. Your podiatrist should prescribe for those on your heels which are often resistant to treatment and for which there may be various causes, such as walking improperly or shoe irritation.

Athlete's foot is a lay term for a fungous infection. Fungi are molds, a household example of which develops on some foods.

I was told a story many years ago by a member of a public relations firm who was present at a conference to promote the sales of an over-the-counter medication for fungous infections of the feet. Sales had been dropping. The group decided on a sales campaign in which the condition would be called policeman's foot.

A few months after the launching of the campaign, another conference was called. The sales had plummeted so badly that the agency feared the loss of the account. The conclusion of the group was that too few people wanted to be identified with policemen!

Then some bright soul suggested that everyone enjoyed being thought of as an athlete. Why not athlete's foot? And thus was born the term that has permeated lay literature and that saved one account for a determined agency!

A fungous infection takes on various forms, affecting most often the areas between the toes, the sole of the foot or the nails. There may be a combination of all these types.

We have, in the previous chapter, discussed the manifestations of fungous infections of the nail.

In fungous involvements of the skin there are sometimes, not always, itching, burning, peeling, cracking, or just dryness. A fungous infection can spread to other parts of the body. Keeping the area dry is important. Fungi thrive in dark, damp places—an environment commonly found in a shoe.

Don't spend your money on over-the-counter sure-cures.

You may, with self-diagnosis, be treating as a fungous infection something that requires completely different treatment. You may, for instance, have psoriasis. Dryness of the skin may be indicative of diabetes.

92

Let your podiatrist or dermatologist make the diagnosis and prescribe for you.

There is a tendency for recurrence of fungous infections in warm weather and in warm climates. While I can offer no statistics, it is my impression that, since the use of air conditioning has become commonplace in homes as well as in offices, fewer patients have bad fungous problems. Certainly, though, it is wise to continue treatment for a few weeks after all the symptoms have disappeared. I also suggest that patients start preventive treatment about May of each year to avoid a flare-up.

Excessive sweating is a major physical and emotional problem for some people. They change hosiery several times a day and ruin shoes because of sogginess. I find that patients will hesitantly mention the excessive sweating, but they almost never mention the putrid odor that sometimes accompanies the sweating. When asked directly, the patient eagerly admits to the odor, grateful for the opportunity to discuss it. He often pours forth a history of the odor being so strong, in spite of cleanliness and frequent hosiery changes, that he hesitates to participate in social activities.

I remember the first time I saw Ralph, who was then a college senior. He was intelligent, attractive and neat. He was consulting me because of an ingrown nail. He was courteous, but obviously restrained in speaking to me.

Because of the macerated appearance of his feet, I picked up one of his socks and shoes. Both were soggy with perspiration. There was an unmistakable odor.

"Do your feet always perspire a great deal?" I asked him.

"Well, yes," he admitted guardedly.

"Is there ever an odor to the perspiration?"

It was as though I had liberated him from bondage! His restraint was gone.

"The odor is awful. Do you smell it now, Dr. Roberts? I washed just before I came here. I always keep an extra pair of socks with me. I change during the day between classes."

Ralph had not gone to an out-of-town college for fear of not having a single room in the dormitory. He shied away from group activities and from spending time with girls.

He admitted he had come to my office only because he could no longer tolerate the pain of his ingrown nail. He had wanted to come sooner, but he had been embarrassed.

He became a star patient. He followed directions explicitly. It was not long before the objectionable odor was well controlled.

That was three years ago. Ralph now has a good position, a worthy challenge for his intelligence.

Two weeks ago I received an invitation to his wedding. A note from him was enclosed. "Please come. I want to say thank-you again."

Sometimes in milder cases of *bromidrosis,* as the disorder breeding the odor is called, the patient is not aware of the odor, but the doctor—and the family—can easily detect it. Many a wife has asked me, "What can I do about my husband's feet? I hate the odor." And just as often the tables are turned with a husband asking for relief from the odor of his wife's feet!

Excessive sweating *(hyperhidrosis)* is not always accompanied by an odor *(bromidrosis).* The sweating may be part of an over-all body reaction in which little

94

can be done to control it on the feet. It may be limited to the hands and feet or to the feet. In these instances helpful regimens and medications can be prescribed.

Bromidrosis stems from improper function of the sweat glands. This may result from faulty foot posture. It can be helped by proper podiatric care and certainly should not be accepted as an albatross to be borne silently. Let your doctor tell you how to control it.

Allergies are always a consideration in prescribing medication. Be sure to tell your doctor of any allergies you know you have.

There is one skin reaction, however, that is sometimes misunderstood by patients. You might have an allergy to adhesive tape, or erroneously think you have such an allergy.

If you do have an allergy to adhesive tape, you'll react to it within hours. On the other hand, if you have adhesive strappings applied periodically over a period of weeks, you may develop a skin irritation simply from the constant contact with the adhesive, combined with the tension of the strapping and with any moisture that develops under the strapping. This is not an allergenic reaction and should not prevent you from using anything from small adhesive strips to large applications of adhesive. Incidentally, such an irritation may not develop on certain people even after months of adhesive tape strappings.

You may have an allergy to the materials used in the construction of a particular pair of shoes. Occasionally a person will be allergic to some material commonly used in almost all shoes. Rubber based adhesives, which are found in most shoes today are often the inciting factor. Any of many other components of the shoe, such as the dyes, the materials used in tanning the leathers or the heel stiffeners, may be the cause.

An allergy to shoes develops as an irritation, sometimes following the contour of a slipper along the top of the toes, the bottom and the sides of the foot. The irritation will appear wherever you have sufficient contact with the shoe for the offending material to take effect.

This type of allergy is known as a contact allergy, since it results from contact with the allergenic substance. Too often, simply because it appears on the foot, the allergy is treated with over-the-counter preparations advertised for a fungous infection. This highlights the need to seek professional care—and when you do, go prepared to give the doctor some idea of how and when the problem began. Were you wearing new or fairly new shoes? Does the irritation subside if you avoid certain shoes for a few days, or is it the same regardless of which shoes you wear?

Your doctor may be able to control the allergy by minimizing the sweating of your feet.

Dr. Alexander A. Fisher is a Clinical Professor of Dermatology at New York University Medical School and an authority on contact dermatitis. He offers the following excellent information if, in spite of treatment for the sweating of your feet, you are allergic to some material generally used in the manufacture of shoes.

Dr. Fisher urges that your doctor determine, if possible, the causative agent of your allergy. Then, with this in mind, you should write to one of the following sources that Dr. Fisher has listed:

. . . McMahan Shoe Store, 429 Peachtree Street, N.E., Atlanta, Georgia 30308 for information where "hypo-allergenic" brown oxford, laced, grain

96

leather shoes for children and women may be obtained in your area.

These shoes are vegetable tanned, free of rubber box toes and contain fish or animal glue or flour paste as rubber cement substitutes.

These shoes are available for all girls and women and for boys up to the age of ten. Julius Altschul, Inc., 117 Grotten Street, Brooklyn, New York, manufactures these shoes.

For "hypo-allergenic" men's and older boys' shoes write to: The Alden Shoe Company, Taunton Street, Middleborough, Massachusetts 02346. This company manufactures the Derma-Pedic shoe for men and the Sable shoe for boys.

The Foot-so-Port Shoe Company, a subsidiary of Musebeck Shoe Company, Inc., Oconomowoc, Wisconsin 53066, will make to order shoes eliminating rubber cements and other materials to which patients show a positive patch test.

The Prescription Footwear Association, whose president is John O. McMahan, P.O. Box 54696, Atlanta, Georgia 30308, is most helpful in obtaining information concerning special shoes for various purposes.

Chapter 9

Keeping in Step as the Years Go By

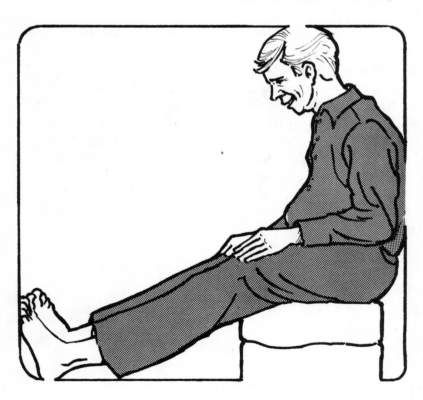

You can make yourself old by being out of step with life around you!

Our society puts a premium on activity even more than on youth. Witness the multitude of advertisements for retirement homes, with the stress always on the variety of activities available—from golf to dancing. Witness the courses preparatory to retirement that are sponsored by an increasing number of large business firms.

The psychologic acceptance of retirement at sixty-five, or even sixty-two, which is in great measure the result of social security and of pension plans, pervades much of the employed population. Retirement for many means being shelved physically and psychologically. Retirement for others means enthusiastic pursuit of a new activity or of an old interest for which there had never been adequate time.

Of one thing you can be sure. If you choose to participate in a satisfying way of life, you must do everything possible to maintain for your body optimum function and optimum comfort.

I would guess, if you're reading this book, that you're

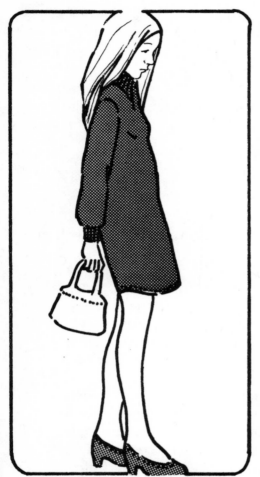

the kind of person who appreciates the importance of your feet not only in walking and in standing and in every other weight bearing activity, but also in contributing to your over-all body health. You can't alter the way your feet function without altering the way the rest of your body functions. You can't have pain in your foot—whether it be caused by a corn, a callus, a bunion, an ingrown nail, a weak arch, a wart or any other painful affliction—without affecting the rest of your body. You automatically withdraw from pain, shifting your weight and throwing the rest of your body out of alignment —your leg, your knee, your thigh, your hip, your abdomen, your spine right up to your head. I have one charming Irish patient who drags into the office periodically. After I have treated her, she invariably stands up and does a jig for me!

If you have arthritis in your feet or in any other part of your body, this is particularly significant. Arthritis is an abnormal condition of the joints. If your feet, the foundation of your body, don't carry your body properly, the bones comprising the joints above your feet cannot be in the correct relationship to each other, and this aggravates the condition.

If you have any circulatory problem—and so many of us do as we get older—remember that good muscle function helps circulation. The muscles have a massaging effect on the blood vessels. Proper use of your feet helps to maintain good muscle function through optimum alignment of your body.

Walking is a great exercise. Your entire body is involved—your feet, your ankles, your legs, your knees, your thighs, your hips, your back, your arms. But who wants to walk if every step is agony? What fun is there in going to that dinner party if you dread putting on your shoes and you wonder how you're going to get through the evening because your feet are bound to ache?

With this in mind, I offer you the first principle for helping yourself stay young. *Remember that your feet are part of your total body.* What happens to your feet affects your body. Much of what happens to your body affects your feet. A stroke, for instance, is an involvement of the arterial supply to the brain, but more often than not it manifests itself in the foot and leg. Another example is an impingement of a spinal nerve causing numbness of the great toe.

Obesity puts additional demands on the feet. Painful feet, however, prevent adequate walking, which, in turn, contributes to obesity. Lower back pain alters gait, but altered gait can cause lower back pain.

The Surgeon General of the United States, in an address to a New York State Podiatry Conference some years ago, highlighted the fundamental importance of foot comfort. He was speaking of nursing homes in which podiatry care was mandatory, not dependent on the request of the patient or the patient's physician. He cited the fact that many patients who had not complained about foot discomfort, but who had spent their time in solitary corners, taking for granted that foot disability was part and parcel of aging, began to walk after they had had podiatry treatment. They emerged from their isolation and joined other patients in the home's activities.

Psychologically the changes were dramatic because of new-found company and new-found interests. Physically the changes were dramatic because the activity enhanced all the body functions. These people ate better. They slept better. Life became more interesting for them.

Thus, the second principle for helping yourself stay young is: Never feel you're too old to try to be comfortable. *Don't accept any discomfort or disability without investigating the cause and possible treatment.* Don't decide that, because you're twenty years older than you were twenty years ago, you should resign yourself to those aches and pains that have come about insidiously.

You would never neglect a fracture or a burn because these happen suddenly and the pain is acute. The majority of the abnormalities of your feet come about gradually, often with discomfort rather than acute pain. By the time the discomfort has advanced to constant pain, you simply forfeit the chances of regaining comfort and function. You reason that this is supposed to happen as you get older. Or perhaps you did see a doctor a few years ago—maybe you consulted several doctors—with no success. Don't give up! Medical thinking may have changed since then. Even if you don't run into a Ponce de Leon, you may find tremendously improved comfort.

One suggestion, if you have no podiatrist, is to ask your local Podiatry Society to give you the names of some doctors in your area. It is likely that such recommendations will lead you to the outstanding doctors in the community. You can locate your local Podiatry Society through your telephone directory or by writing to the American Podiatry Association, 20 Chevy Chase Circle, N.W., Washington, D.C. 20015. Incidentally, if you do write to the American Podiatry Association, you might also ask that you be sent any pamphlets they have on geriatrics. These pamphlets are pertinent and informative.

The third principle for helping yourself stay young is: *Use your body.*

As youngsters we run and climb and bend and stretch, using our whole bodies in play and in school physical training classes. Many of us develop athletic skills such as skating and horseback riding. Some become valuable members of athletic teams, ranging from football to rowing crew to tennis.

By the time we reach our twenties and thirties the demands of earning a living and caring for a family diminish our time for "body-using" activities. By the fifties too many of us set as our goal "*protecting my body*" rather than "*using* my body." By the sixties many of us unquestioningly accept an inability to use our bodies beyond the basic needs of daily activity.

Unless there is a specific medical reason for avoiding real motion, don't cop out on agility. Don't hesitate to bend and stretch and walk, even though it hurts a bit at the outset. Try to pick up that paper from the floor by bending your knees in a squatting position. Make that bed by really stretching across to the other side to straighten the blanket. Put on your most comfortable shoes and walk to the movie instead of taking the car. And, while you're walking, let your arms swing along in rhythm with your legs. Keep the light chain in the clothes closet short enough that you must really stretch to reach it. Use your ingenuity to think of other ways to force yourself to use your body for routine chores.

We can get older in any or all of three ways— chronologically, psychologically, and physically.

For each year we get older chronologically we should not only add a gay birthday candle, but have a wow of a celebration! Would you be around to read this if you hadn't become chronologically older on your last birthday?

Psychologically we become older for unfortunate reasons too numerous to be discussed here. If you are psychologically old you will find it difficult to accept the three principles I am urging upon you:

1. Remember that your feet are part of your total body.

2. Don't accept any discomfort or disability without investigating the cause and possible treatment.

3. Use your body.

People who have grown psychologically old will simply answer, "That all sounds find, but it's not for me. She doesn't know the troubles I have!"

Remember Dr. Coué who used to say, "Day by day in every way I am getting better and better"? It's not all rubbish. Simply by deciding you can, you've taken the first step toward achieving more than you have up to now.

"Slowing the Clock of Age," an article by Rona Cherry and Laurence Cherry that appeared in the *New York Times Magazine,* discussed the theories of the biochemistry of the aging process. In speaking of organizations such as the American Association of Retired Persons they quoted Margaret Clark of Langley-Porter Neuropsychiatric Institute:

> These older people's organizations are beginning to have an impact on the terribly negative self-image most older people have. Older people are starting to accept not only themselves, but also other older people . . . you find old people who say, "I can't stand being with old people." That's beginning to change. Older people are looking at one another and saying, "Hey, you're not so bad after all."

Physically, as we get older, changes take place within our bodies on a much less rigid timetable than exists in early life. Apparently, much depends upon our genes and on the physical and psychologic stresses of our way of life.

In examining a sixty-year-old patient, any doctor will look for conditions that he would not expect to find in the twenty-year-old. (This is the reason every doctor asks your age and is turned off by the patient who answers, "Over twenty-one!")

Among the systemic disorders particularly significant to the podiatrist are:

arthritis
diabetes

neurologic problems
arteriosclerosis (hardening of the arteries)
other circulatory deficiencies
any history of circulatory involvements such as
    phlebitis
    Buerger's disease
    intermittent claudication
    varicose veins

He will also ask about any history of:

bone changes like osteoporosis
spinal column problems as a compressed disc or
                nerve impingements
knee problems
fractures

Some of the symptoms the podiatrist may well expect
to find in the older patient, in addition to corns and
callus, are:

lower back pain
cramping of the feet and/or legs, particularly at
            night   .
dryness of the skin
gait changes
decreased sensitivity to pain, touch or heat
fatigue on walking
coldness of the feet
swelling of the ankles and/or feet

He will look for:

ulcerations
fungous conditions of the skin and/or nails

    fissures (cracks), particularly of the heels
    ingrown nails
    bunions

As you read down these lists, you may be saying, "There I am!" The lists simply reinforce the premise that your feet are part of your total body, that what affects your body affects your feet.

Circulatory deficiency requires special attention to the feet, since any injury or neglect may result in ulceration or even gangrene. Every diabetic patient knows the importance of foot care to avoid gangrene and possible amputation.

An impingement on a nerve, possibly because of a compressed disc, may cause numbness of the foot. A knee problem or an old fracture may cause faulty walking, often putting undue strain on the "good" foot.

I refer you to the more detailed sections in this book on arthritis, diabetes and various other ailments affecting the feet.

The list of symptoms, such as decreased sensitivity to pain, touch or heat, dryness of the skin and coldness of the feet again echo the concept that your general body health affects your feet. Lower back pain, cramping, fatigue and swelling often result from a foot condition and demonstrate the effect of the feet on other parts of your body.

Don't accept disability or discomfort without investigating the cause and possible treatment. Even if your arthritis or circulatory condition can't be cured, the probability is that your foot comfort and function can be improved and the chances of catastrophic complications can be avoided.

There is some erosion of the fat pads of the foot as we grow older. The skin tends to become dry. Fissures often develop on the heels and can be very painful. It is wise to use a lubricant routinely. The residue of a face moisturizer that a woman has left on her hands can well be used on the feet. A vegetable shortening is an inexpensive and excellent lubricant. This, of course, could be bought in a grocery store or supermarket. Your podiatrist may have his own preference among creams and lotions. Speak to him about this.

Use your body. Those of you with some relatively incapacitating conditions will rightly ask, "How? I'm not supposed to exert myself." It is for you, in particular, that I stress the following foot and leg exercises. These exercises will get the "motor turning over" in the morning and will offer relaxation at night.

The exercises are done in bed before you get up in the morning and again in bed at night. Don't exercise to the point of fatigue. Tomorrow you'll be able to do more. If you start with just once for each movement, tomorrow you'll be able to do it two or three or four times!

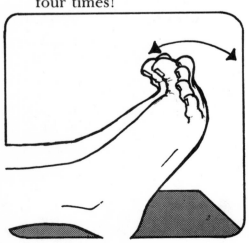

1. Lying in bed, bend your toes down and then up. Do it deliberately, not just flapping in the wind.

2. The second exercise consists simply

of making a circle with the right foot in counter-clock wise direction. All the motion should be at the ankle, not at the knee or hip. Do it slowly and deliberately. Then do the same with the left foot, but in a clockwise direction. In each case the beginning of your circle is in the direction of the midline of the body.

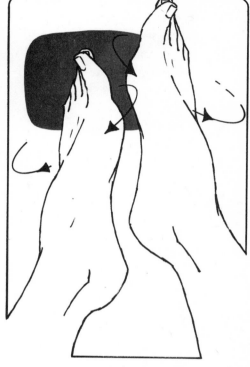

3. The third exercise is just bending your knee (even though it may make a grating noise in the process) as you lie on your back. Grasp your leg with both hands and gently pull your knee back towards your body.

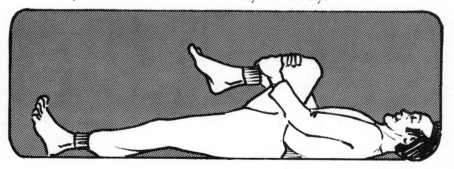

You'll be surprised at how much easier these exercises will be within a week, and how much more agile you'll be—if you start today. It's getting started that's so often a hurdle. What do you say? Tonight and then again tomorrow morning?

Chapter **10**

How Does Your General
Health Affect Your Feet?

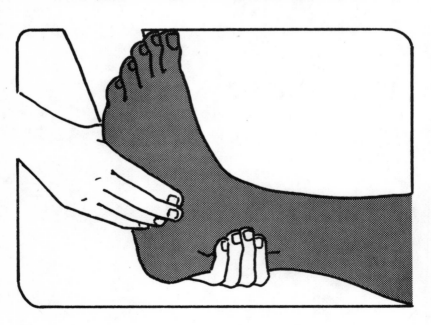

The first indication of systemic disease is often found in the feet.

This has given rise to some valid therapies as well as various fads and theories.

Dr. M. W. Locke of Williamsburg, Ontario in Canada, based his entire practice on his belief that, "Nobody can feel well if his feet are sick."

In the 1930s thousands of people came from very distant points to be treated by Dr. Locke, whose therapy was manipulation of the feet. These people came because of his reputation for helping patients with ailments such as synovitis, neuritis, sciatica and arthritis. Rex Beach in his book, *The Hands of Dr. Locke,* records a conversation between Dr. Locke and a patient who had come to him with an arthritic shoulder.

Instead of examining the affected part he treated her arches, whereupon she protested.

"But, doctor! It isn't my foot that hurts. It's my shoulder."

With a twinkle in his . . . eyes, he replied, "I know. But if you step on a dog's tail, which end of him yelps?"

I have no desire to evaluate Dr. Locke's therapeutic procedure. I do believe, however, that improper foot posture with the resulting strain on the body and interference with optimum circulation and metabolism, will not only aggravate existing arthritis and related conditions, but will make people who are predisposed to these conditions more likely to get them.

Witness the fact that many patients are referred to podiatrists not because of foot symptoms, but rather because of lower back pain, knee pain or extreme fatigue after walking or standing.

More recently we have been hearing of reflexology, or zone therapy, a method of applying pressure to charted areas of the foot. Each spot apparently has "nerve connections" or "energy connections" to some specific part of the body. The therapeutic effect of this pressure is attributed possibly to improved circulation.

Essentially the premise is that any part of the body can be beneficially stimulated through the feet. Again, I am in no position—nor do I have the desire—to pass judgment on reflexology, which has, in the literature that I have read, been presented on a nonmedical basis.

Within the foot are several points used in acupuncture therapy to treat disorders in parts of the body that are distant from the foot, including toothache, backache and abdominal pain. We of the Western world are still in the process of learning about and of evaluating acupuncture. At this writing I can say no more than that I have been tremendously impressed with what patients have told me of the lessening or disappearance of long-standing subjective symptoms such as pain.

The feet reveal the early signs of many systemic

diseases, and they are often seriously affected by these diseases.

Let's consider the effect of some common systemic diseases on the feet.

If you have diabetes, your physician has probably alerted you to the importance of continuing foot care as a protective measure. The purpose is to avoid, rather than try to cure, conditions that may, in the extreme, result in gangrene. When you hear of an amputation on a diabetic patient, it almost invariably involves a foot or a foot and leg. The reason is that most diabetics develop circulatory problems. The circulation of the foot and leg is the most vulnerable in the entire body. The blood supply is the least good, and so it is the site of the greatest incidence of gangrene.

The foot often reveals the first symptoms of diabetes—abrasions or ulcers that do not heal, dry, brittle nails, dry skin, tingling or numbness.

Ulcers are breaks in the tissue that lead to disintegration of underlying tissues and may become progressively larger and deeper. You may be more familiar with stomach, duodenal, or intestinal ulcers, which are breaks in the tissues within the body. The ulcers of which we are speaking appear in the skin and tissues immediately underlying the skin. They appear frequently on the feet of a diabetic at sites of irritation or injury. Healing is slow even when the patient is "under control" through medication, diet or other care his physician has prescribed. Ulcers can occur under a nail, either because of improvident cutting of the nail by the patient, because of pressure from shoes or because of an injury such as something falling on the toe.

Ulcers develop most often on the ball of the foot,

either because of a patient's attempt at "home surgery" or because of faulty patterns in walking and
standing. The constant minute injuries, caused by
banging down improperly on the foot with each step
can equal the impact of a single severe injury.

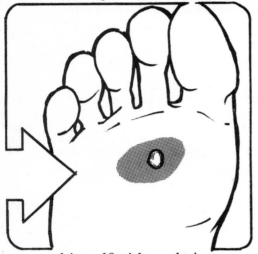

Sometimes ulcers on
the foot are the result of
neglecting either a corn
or callus, which eventu-
ally brings so much pres-
sure against the foot that
it breaks down the un-
derlying tissues.

A very great hazard
for the diabetic is the
eventual decrease in sen-
sory, pain, and temper-
ature perception. This
permits him to injure
himself without being aware of it and subsequently to
neglect the injury, aggravating the problem.

Mr. Rodman, a diabetic, is an example of this. He
was conscientious about seeing me once a month and
he came in one summer day for his regular appointment.

I was aghast when I saw the bottom of his right foot.
There, imbedded very deeply in the tissue, was a splinter fully a half inch long. The entire area around the
splinter was badly inflamed.

He had felt no pain. He had no idea of how he had
gotten the splinter—until he recalled having walked
barefooted on a beach at a place where there was a lot
of seawood and driftwood lying about.

Fortunately he had had his routine appointment.

116

The splinter was removed and the damaged tissue eventually healed. And Mr. Rodman was saved from perhaps a major disaster.

Yet, with all of these very real dangers, a diabetic can be grateful for today's advances in knowledge and in therapy, for they can help him to lead a satisfying, active life.

If any of your blood relatives is a diabetic, you're lax, to put it mildly, if you don't go to your physician for periodic blood examinations to determine whether or not you have diabetes. Most doctors suggest annual examinations. I urge an examination every six months. A whole year is a long time—lots of things can develop in a year.

The following are imperative foot care cautions for you if you're diabetic. Neglecting any one of them might spell disaster for you.

1. Examine your feet daily for any abrasions or abnormality.

2. Don't "treat" your own feet. You shouldn't even cut your own nails, let alone your corns or callus. You should visit your podiatrist on a time, not a pain, basis. The average time interval is one month, but this should be the determination of your podiatrist.

3. Don't use any over-the-counter medications on your feet unless they are prescribed for you. They frequently cause ulcers even on the feet of people with no circulatory problems.

4. Your feet should be bathed daily in comfortably warm, *not hot,* water. Dry your feet well, but gently, *including the areas between the toes.*

5. Use a lubricant on your feet morning and night to keep the skin soft. A moisturizer, a vegetable shortening, or a body cream can be used.

6. If your feet perspire excessively, ask your podiatrist to prescribe a safe powder.

7. Your shoes must be of soft leather or fabric. Reptiles and plastics lack porosity and flexibility. Your shoes must fit with no area of irritation. This may involve treatment of your feet to maintain them in the correct weightbearing position.

8. Don't use circular garters.

9. Don't wear socks with an excessively tight top band.

10. Don't wear "support" hosiery, because it may constrict the foot. Be sure your hosiery is an easy fit. Poorly fitting hosiery can be as harmful as poorly fitting shoes.

11. Don't mend your hosiery. You can't afford to walk on anything that may irritate your feet.

12. Avoid adhesive tape, which may irritate or tear your skin. In a pharmacy you can buy extremely effective substitutes for adhesive tape. They are hypo-allergenic and easy to remove from the skin, even from a hairy surface.

13. Avoid constricting boots. Women's high, tight-legged boots are particularly suspect of causing circulatory problems, such as phlebitis, even in the non-diabetic.

118

14. Don't—don't—use a heating pad or hot water bottle. Your perception of heat may not be accurate. At night you may want to wear socks in bed. If the entire room is cold, try using a safe electric room heater with a thermostat.

15. Don't smoke.

If you are not diabetic, but have hardening of the arteries (arteriosclerosis), Buerger's disease (*thromboangiitis obliterans*), Raynaud's disease (gangrene), or any other occlusive arterial disease, the fifteen preventive admonitions apply to you, too.

One of the first symptoms of some circulatory diseases may be intermittent claudication. "Claudication" is derived from the Latin word *claudicare* which means "to limp." The person with claudication is able to walk only a certain distance before he feels pain in the calf muscles. He has no choice but to stop. After two or three minutes of resting he can start walking again. Eventually, as the blood supply to the feet and legs becomes more impaired, the distance he is able to walk before the onset of pain decreases.

Other systemic conditions may be accompanied by alterations in the circulation to the feet and legs, among them cardiac disease, hyperthyroidism, kidney disease and pernicious anemia.

Mrs. Lewis was a department store saleswoman. She had cut her own nails, going deeply into the nail groove of her great toe. When, two weeks later, the pain and inflammation continued, she consulted me.

Mrs. Lewis apparently was a healthy woman in her fifties with no history of disease beyond a cold. Her toe, however, did not heal.

I began to suspect diabetes or some other problem.

I sent her for a whole battery of tests. The report came back—leukemia.

The following quotation from the *Journal of Podiatric Education* (March, 1973) lends emphasis to the effect of one's general health on the feet.

In a recent survey involving the Harlem community, several thousand children, selected on a statistically valid random sampling basis, were examined in the clinics of the New York College of Podiatric Medicine. Two cases of sickle-cell anemia were detected. Sickle-cell anemia has a propensity to produce ankle ulcers, which are often first detected during podiatric examinations. (The podiatrist, therefore, is often the first practitioner to recognize undetected sickle-cell anemia, by the presence of these ulcers.) Thirteen children were found to have a secondary syphilis. (Similarly, secondary syphilis is often first recognized by the podiatrist by the presence of small cornlike lesions on the soles or the palms.) These patients were immediately referred to the Department of Health for proper treatment. This early recognition of syphilis. . . often prevents serious sequelae of blindness, neurological damage, or death.

A stroke, as you well know, can paralyze a foot and leg with resulting ulcers due to pressure of shoes or of braces and with wasting of the foot and leg muscles from lack of use.

Abnormalities in the vertebral column, such as a compressed disc, or in the spinal cord, such as a tumor, may cause numbness or tingling in the foot (often in the great toe), loss of sensation, and diminished motion and loss of strength in the foot. Very frequently the first symptoms are in the feet.

The nails often betray systemic disease. Dr. Milton Ashur of Jersey City has detailed these changes well in Weinstein's *Principles and Practice of Podiatry.*

Heart and lung disease and circulatory conditions may be accompanied by coarse nails that curve over the enlarged ends of the toes.

Nails which are concave like a spoon are often found in patients with anemia, hyperthyroidism, hypothyroidism or syphilis. If your nails are spoon nails, however, don't despair on the spot. They also occur as congenital defects.

Scarlet fever, syphilis or leprosy may cause the complete loss of the nails.

There may be alternate transverse ridges and grooves in the nails resulting from vitamin deficiencies. This is frequently true of alcoholics.

Medications containing silver may give the nail a slate-blue color. Gold therapy will turn the nails a brown-black, as will mercury taken internally.

Now, in spite of this information about nails, don't become your own diagnostician, convinced that dire things are happening within your body. Maybe your body is behaving just fine and there is a perfectly good explanation for the appearance of your nails. Just use the information as a basis for getting professional advice.

Various drug reactions show themselves in the feet. Penicillin, for instance, may cause a dry peeling of the skin.

Heroin addicts often have foot tremors. In fact, at one center in New York City every heroin user's feet are examined because most of the patients with marked foot tremors are long-term or heavy users of heroin.

Swelling of the feet and ankles may be due to a tumor in the abdominal area, an abnormality of the kidneys or of the heart, varicose veins, cirrhosis of the liver or a vitamin deficiency. There are numerous other reasons for swelling of the feet and legs, ranging from premenstrual swelling to a local injury. Incidentally, oral contraceptives sometimes are the cause.

Frequently diuretics (medications to increase urination) are prescribed to reduce such swelling. It would seem desirable, however, to search for the actual cause, rather than depend on medication to eliminate the symptom temporarily.

There are two areas on the foot that are often mis-

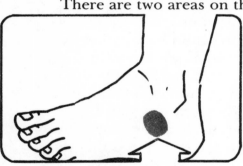

taken for swellings. One is on the top of the foot toward the outer side and just in front of the ankle. It is a muscle that is normally found there. In some people it is more prominent than in others. If you want to verify that it is a muscle, not a swelling, wiggle your toes up and down. If it's a muscle, it will move as it contracts and relaxes.

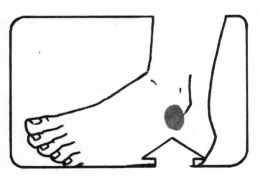

The other area mistaken often, very often, for a swelling appears below and in front of the outer ankle bone of some women. It's simply a fat pad that develops in many women in their forties and fifties. The size of the fat pad remains constant. If it were a swelling, it would sometimes be larger, sometimes smaller.

I could cite many additional examples of systemic disease symptoms that appear in the foot or in the foot and leg. My purpose is not to detail an entire medical course, nor do I want to frighten you into an orgy of self-diagnosis. I simply want to highlight the inseparable unity of the feet with the rest of the body and to impress upon you the necessity of investigating symptoms. The swelling may be due not to a tumor, but to the fact that it is a hot, humid summer day! Why not make sure?

Obesity is one great bugaboo that confronts too many of us—and it has serious repercussions in our feet. You certainly don't have to look to your feet for the diagnosis of obesity. Just look in your mirror. It is obvious that the bones and muscles and tendons and ligaments of feet that should be carrying 125 pounds are going to be overworked, perhaps beyond the point of tolerance, if they must carry 200 pounds!

The foot is a frequent site for arthritis. Many of us have arthritis in other parts of our bodies. Since the joints are involved, it is apparent that, if the feet are not maintaining the body in the correct position, the joints above the feet will tend to be in less than the optimum position. For example, improving the position and function of the feet will not eliminate the arthritis of the spine, but it may decrease pain in the spine. Neglecting the position and function of the feet may aggravate the arthritic condition.

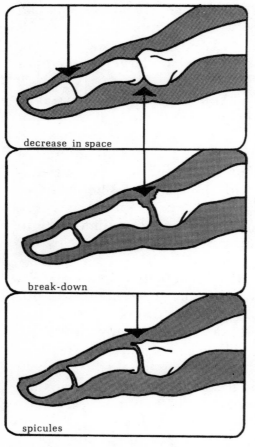

decrease in space

break-down

spicules

Arthritis is a condition involving the joints of the body. Various abnormalities might exist within a joint—a decrease in the space between bones, an increase in the space, a breakdown of part of the bone, a growth of spicules of bone.

Gout is a form of arthritis. It may appear in various joints in the body, but perhaps the most frequent site is the great toe joint. The cause is a chemical imbalance in the body which generates excess production of uric acid. If you have gout, you know the excruciating pain of an attack and you may well agree with Dr. Thomas Sydenham's description in 1683 of an acute attack, drawn from personal experience:

The victim goes to bed and sleeps in good health. About two o'clock in the morning he is awakened by a severe pain in the great toe; more rarely in the heel, ankle or instep. This pain is like that of a dislocation, and yet the parts feel as if cold water were poured over them. Then follow chills and shivers, and a little fever. The pain, which was at first moderate, becomes more intense. With its intensity the chills and shivers increase. After a time this comes to its height . . . now it is a gnawing pain, and a pressure and tightening. So exquisite and lively meanwhile is the feeling of the part affected, that it cannot bear the weight of the bedclothes nor the jar of a person walking in the room. The night is passed in torture, sleeplessness, turning of the part affected, and perpetual change of posture.

Obviously, in addition to any medication prescribed for the chemical imbalance, a gouty joint should be protected from unnecessary injury, such as constantly banging down on the great toe joint in walking and standing.

You and I know the far-reaching effect of emotional upheavals on the body. We know, for instance, that an emotional maladjustment is often the fundamental reason for obesity. We know, too, how much better our entire bodies feel after a happy experience.

Extreme emotional problems can cause truly dramatic symptoms in the feet and legs—even loss of function or paralysis. Anyone with diabetes or gout or rheumatoid arthritis knows that a bad emotional episode can trigger an attack.

At times a patient who has shown consistent improvement suddenly complains of pains he's not had for several weeks or of brand new pains. I am as anxious as he is to track down the cause of the apparent backslide. If the physical condition gives no clues, I always ask whether there has been a particularly upsetting incident since the patient's last visit. The chances are that the answer is yes, but only the more psychologically oriented patients recognize the connection.

Some of the answers I've gotten are: "My son telephoned me to say he's getting a divorce." "My boss is retiring and I may not have a job." "My mother-in-law is coming to live with me."

Most of us have experienced a distressing situation that left us "tired." It may have been strictly emotional, but it surely did result in physical fatigue—often with the comment, "I could hardly drag my feet!"

Chapter **11**

Find More Comfort in the Shoes You Buy

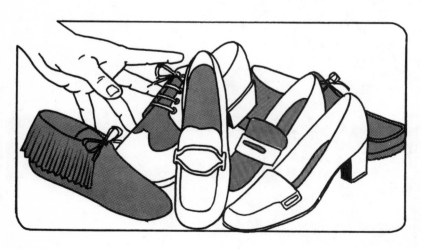

The long red shoehorn that I bought in Norway has inscribed on it *Den vet best hvor skoen trykker, som har den pa.* It means, "He who wears the shoe best knows where it pinches."

While there may be some philosophical implication in this, obviously we Americans are not alone in suffering through one pair of shoes after another. But, although he might know where it pinches, the wearer seldom knows *why* it pinches—and why every other shoe he buys eventually pinches or just downright hurts.

If you can't find comfortable shoes, it may be due primarily to your feet and only secondarily to the shoes.

I certainly hold no brief for shoe styling and for shoe merchandising. Shoe styles, particularly women's, change seasonally, but feet don't. Shoes are sold in pairs, but no one has a pair of feet. One foot is always larger than the other. Your two feet are no more identical than the two sides of your face. If the consumer's health were the chief consideration, shoes would be sold as right shoes and left shoes. This, however, would lead to additional inventory problems that apparently no manufacturer or merchant is willing to take upon himself.

Shoe salesmen SELL shoes. They should FIT shoes. They are not Machiavellian. They simply have no source for learning how to fit a shoe. There are a few men and women who, by experience, have learned a great deal about shoe fitting, but they certainly are in the minority.

But you, moreover, may be guilty of encouraging a shoe salesman to sell you a pair of poorly fitting shoes. A man knows that every style of suit will not fit him, regardless of size. A woman knows that some styles in dresses will look dreadful on her, regardless of size. But, somehow, few people realize that some shoe styles just won't fit their feet. I am not referring to extremes in heels or pointed toes. Some basic styles just won't fit some feet, no matter how attractive they may look in the store window.

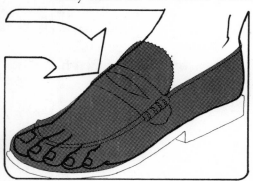

A good example is the loafer with a high tongue on a foot with a prominent area over the arch. The chances are that the tongue will cause pressure on the bones that form the prominence. Another example is the shoe that tapers even conservatively on a foot that is quite rectangular in shape. Too many people select shoes for their eyes, not for their feet. They tell the shoe salesman what they want and then are adamant in their choice, even if he suggests a better fitting shoe.

Many people are equally adamant about their shoe sizes. Simply asking for a 7B shoe every time you buy shoes is ridiculous. How many of us always take the same size in a suit or a dress? The size varies with the style and with the manufacturer. In certain shoes the "7B foot" may do better in a 6½C or in a 7½A.

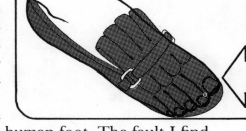

Too many shoes seem not to be shaped for the human foot. The fault I find most frequently in the way shoes are fitted is in the width. Sometimes this is because of the pur-chaser's insistence or lack of knowledge. Often the fifth toe—or the fourth and fifth toes— are actually jammed against the side of the shoe, and the great toe is pushed over to the center of the toe-box. If the front of the shoe is wide enough for the foot to be resting on the sole, frequently the heel fit is far too roomy.

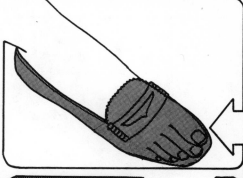

A woman's open-toe and open-heel shoe with an instep strap has two great virtues. The first is that there is no wall against which the toes hit. The second is that

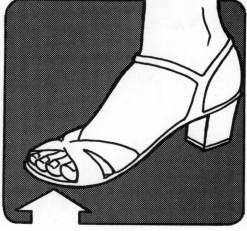

131

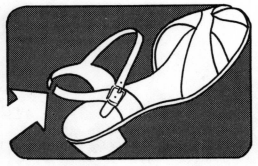

the heel fit becomes little or no problem and hence the shoe can be fitted wide enough for the front part of the foot to be resting on the bottom of the shoe with no toes squeezed up on the sides. If the heel strap is too loose, it is easy to have a shoe cobbler remove a piece from the strap, reseaming it to the proper size, just as one would have the seam of a dress or suit taken in.

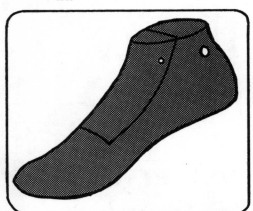

Some people erroneously believe that a foot will "spread" in a shoe that is adequately wide. This, of course, is fallacious reasoning. Does your hand become wider because you wear a glove that is comfortable and does not "squeeze" —or because you wear no glove at all?

A shoe last is the wooden reproduction of the approximate shape of the human foot. The shoe is made over this wooden last. Harold J. Quimby, in his "Pacemakers of Progress" speaks of three kinds of lasts:

A standard or normal last "designed to fit the average foot."

A combination or slender heel last designed to provide "a snug fit throughout the back part of the foot yet providing ample room for the toes and across the ball of the foot. . . . Combination lasts are usually made for the construction of better grade shoes!" Shoes made on combination lasts generally have two width markings separated by a slash as A/C. This indicates an A width in the areas of the instep and heel of the shoe and a C width across the front of the shoe.

An orthopedic last which Mr. Quimby defines necessarily vaguely as a last for shoes "which . . . aid walking and provide a greater measure of comfort for structurally weak feet."

Let me stress that anyone whose foot condition prompts him to think in terms of an "orthopedic last" should not go near a shoe store until he has consulted his podiatrist to find out first what care and second what shoes his feet need.

The difference in length of a shoe from one size to the next within the same width is $1/3$ of an inch. Thus size 8B would be $1/3$ of an inch longer than size 7B and $1/6$ of an inch longer than size $7\frac{1}{2}$B. There is a difference of $1/16$ to $1/8$ of an inch from one width to the next.

While some shoes are clearly marked numerically for length and alphabetically for width, as $8\frac{1}{2}$C, others are marked in a code. The first letter of the code is the numerical counterpart of the alphabetical width.

Thus:

> 0 indicates AA
> 1 indicates A
> 2 indicates B
> 3 indicates C
> 4 indicates D
> 5 indicates E
> 6 indicates EE

The second number represents the size. If the final number is zero, the shoe size is a full size. If the final number is 5, the shoe is a half size. Thus:

> 175 indicates $7\frac{1}{2}$A
> 4110 indicates 11D
> 685 indicates $8\frac{1}{2}$EE

Less expensive shoes, which are generally of cheaper construction, are often sold in widths of S (slim), N (narrow), M (medium), and W (wide). This means the shoe store must have less inventory in size ranges, and you have less chance of an adequate fit than in shoes with a greater range of widths.

The less expensive the shoe, the more frequently there is a lack of uniformity in sizes. Even more expensive shoes have some variation in fit, but they are kept on the last for a longer time so that they mold to fit more accurately. Shoes of better construction can usually be used longer, retaining the original fitting qualities for most of the life of the shoes. These qualities are quickly lost in cheaper shoes.

Even custom-made shoes vary in uniformity of size. This is the reason that one firm imprints a number on the face of the heel block of each custom-made shoe. It is not the style number, but the identification number of the man who has pulled the leather over the last. 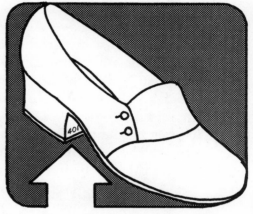 The theory is that some men will pull the leather more firmly than others. The identification number permits the buyer to have the same man work on the second pair of shoes.

Inexpensive shoes are often blatantly advertised as cure-alls. Recently in the *New York Times* a shoe store advertised:

Hammer toes? Our "barefoot classic" . . . comfortable, good-looking . . . and a great walker. Sheer perfection for those crowded toes. Have it in black, brown or navy suede. Sizes 4 to 11 M, W. . . .

This store is probably typical of the kind with inexperienced help who will ask "What size do you take?", rather than measure your feet.

Don't let an attractive picture of a shoe in an advertisement guide your choice. Chances are, it looks better than it is. The commercial artist is paid to make the product look attractive, not necessarily realistic.

The softer, more flexible the uppers (all of the shoe above the sole), the easier it is to wear the shoe.

135

Suedes are easier to wear than heavy leathers. Fabrics, as in sneakers, have the flexibility to minimize foot irritation. Plastics, lacking flexibility and porosity, are among the more undesirable shoe materials. This is true also of reptiles with the exception of snake skin which is extremely soft. Cordovan is heavy and unyielding. Synthetics have little or no "give." Patent leather lacks porosity and has far less flexibility than many other leathers, although the crinkle patent leather that has been fashionable recently is more flexible than other patent leather.

Leather soles offer greater porosity than do synthetics. Rubber soles and ripple soles are extremely comfortable. They give resiliency to each step. They may, however, increase the degree of perspiration in people who already have a problem with foot perspiration or foot odor. While these soles provide less support for the foot, this probably is no consideration for you unless you need some professional foot care anyway. Even if this is so, with adequate modification the shoes may be extremely comfortable.

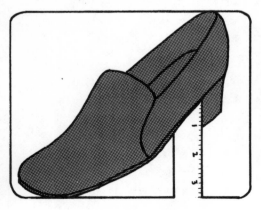

When a shoe salesman speaks of an 8/8 heel, he means a heel one inch high, measured vertically along the front surface of the heel from the bottom of the heel to the point where it joins the shoe proper. Heels are measured in eighths of an inch. Thus, a 12/8 heel is 1½ inches high.

Rubber heel lifts buffer the impact of the foot coming down on hard surfaces far better than do leather lifts. Lifts of synthetic materials, while they last longer than rubber lifts, are less yielding and often so smooth that there is danger of slipping.

Shoes must be selected with a specific function in mind. What might serve as a "scotch-and-soda" or "Sunday-go-to-meeting" shoe for a few hours during a week shouldn't be relegated to an "everyday-go-to-work" shoe when it becomes shabby. Would you wear your tuxedo to the office just because it no longer looked elegant enough for the next formal dinner? Would you wear your cocktail dress to do the marketing because it was time to buy a new cocktail dress? Actually, if you did, you'd suffer less physical harm than you might by wearing dress-up shoes for everyday occasions. Remember that your shoe is the only article of clothing in your wardrobe whose fit can do permanent injury to your body!

High heels, or at least higher heels, are generally a woman's choice for dressy occasions. They may be less comfortable than a lower heel when worn just for dress-up, but high heels are less detrimental when worn occasionally than when they are worn all the time. Those of you who always wear high heels know the difficulty of walking in low-heeled shoes, even though the balls of your feet may ache in the shoes with high heels. This is what has happened. Normally our muscles permit us to walk with our heels flat on the ground, as man did in walking barefoot, before shoes were invented. When a high heel is worn the body is thrust forward. To compensate for this, the abdomen protrudes and the back curves in. Eventually the muscles in the back of the leg shorten and the body maintains this swayback position.

At this point, if lower heels are worn, they cause pull on the now-shorter muscles in the back of the leg and make the wearer feel as though she is falling backwards.

If a woman limits the use of high heels to special occasions, and wears shoes with lower heels most of the time, the muscle shortening does not occur.

When you buy a pair of shoes, having decided on its purpose, you might have the unique good fortune to know a salesman on whose judgment you can rely. If you must depend on your own judgment, here are a few guidelines:

1. Decide on the use to which you will put the shoes.

2. Shop for your shoes late in the day, after you've been on your feet for awhile. Your feet may be larger then than they were earlier in the day.

3. Remember that in warmer weather your feet may swell. Allow for this even though you spend most of your time in air-conditioned buildings.

4. If the shoe salesman simply asks you your size, take yourself to another shoe store.

   Each foot should be measured, since there always is some variance in size. Of course, the larger foot is the one that should govern size selection. Even a weight bearing measuring device, however, gives the shoe salesman no absolutely specific information. The measuring device is two dimensional; your foot is three dimensional. The device will give the minimum length, not the optimum length. It will give only a general idea of width.

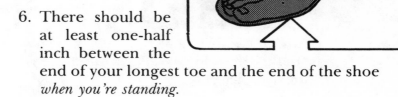

5. The widest part of your foot should fit the widest part of the shoe, not just a bit in front of or behind it.

6. There should be at least one-half inch between the end of your longest toe and the end of the shoe *when you're standing.*

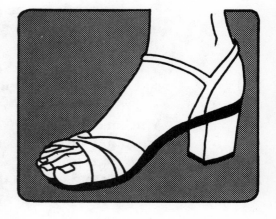

Your longest toe is not necessarily your great toe. It may be your second or even your third toe. In an open-toe shoe your longest toe should be well within the shoe, not dangling out like a blackboard pointer.

7. The heel should fit snugly.

The heel strap of an open-back shoe can be reseamed, making for a more snug fit. This, of course, is why an open-toe and open-back shoe is *the* choice woman's shoe.

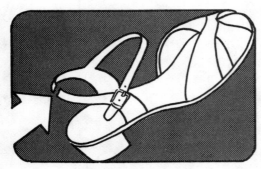

The most desirable type of open-heel shoe has an instep strap that consists of not one piece that encircles the ankle, but two pieces, each of which has its own function. The back piece holds the rear part of the shoe in place. The front piece serves as the shoe clasp.

Simply tightening the front strap does not make the back strap tighter.

8. Your feet are largest when you're standing squarely with your full weight on them.

You can wiggle your toes even in a shoe that is much too small for you. That is no real test for fit or comfort. Test shoes by standing first on one foot and then on the other. Be sure to stand *and* walk in new shoes in the shoe store.

140

9. While you're standing, the leather or fabric of the front of the shoe should be able to be rippled slightly as a finger is rolled over it from side to side.

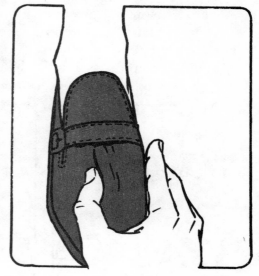

10. When you stand there should be enough depth from the top to the sole for your toes not to hit against the top of the shoe.

In women's shoes, particularly, the top of the shoe often tapers down to almost no space at the front tip, crushing the toes from top to bottom.

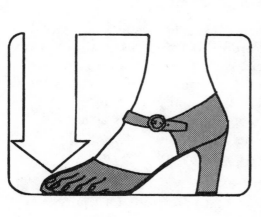 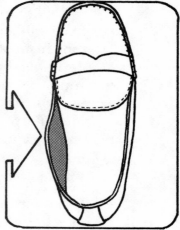

11. There is no such thing as an "arch" shoe.

    Some shoes have a long counter, which means that the stiffening around the back of the shoe extends forward along the side. This long counter is readily broken down by a foot that rolls to the inner side.

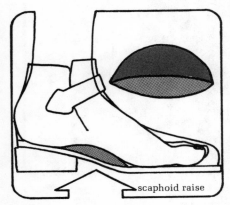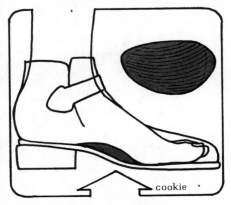

scaphoid raise

cookie

12. Don't let a shoe salesman put a metatarsal pad or a cookie (a concave shell at the arch area) or a scaphoid raise (a convex rubber raise at the arch area) into your shoes.

    Even a filler (material, such as felt, to keep your foot from slipping forward in the shoe) is undesirable because it decreases the space for your foot and does nothing to position your foot properly. A filler might be acceptable for one of a pair of shoes if there is a marked discrepancy in the size of your two feet. The filler might improve the fit of the shoe on your smaller foot.

    It is interesting that your podiatrist, after years of schooling, must examine your feet to know what treatment you require, but the shoe salesman, by some divine decree, just glances at your feet and—zoomie!—he has all the answers.

In the first place, one part of the foot cannot be altered without considering the rest of the

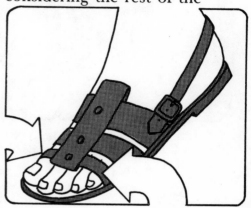

foot. Secondly, a very fundamental condition, as a circulatory problem or a nerve impingement, may be overlooked while you're experimenting with the shoe man's panaceas.

13. If you're buying a sandal, be sure the straps don't irritate your fifth toe or your great toe joint.

14. Run your hand along the entire inside of the shoe to be sure there are no wrinkles, loose linings, lasting tacks, ridges between the inner sole and the sides of the shoes, or any other irregularities.

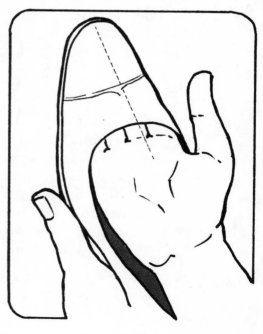

15. Be sure the stitching of any decora-

143

tive pattern does not go to the inside of the shoe, creating a ridge or bulk to irritate the foot.

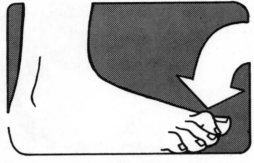

16. If you have a hammertoe, be sure no seam is over that toe.

17. If you wear arch supports or moulds, take them along with you when you go shoe-shopping so that they can be inserted into the shoes before you try them on.

18. And—if you're satisfied on all these scores —before you pay for the shoes, have the salesman verify that, if they are uncomfortable when you try them at home you can return them for a refund, *providing they are perfectly clean.*

Your feet never really settle into new shoes in the short time you're in a shoe store.

Any responsible store will agree to refund your money, not simply to exchange the shoes. What if these shoes are not comfortable and there are no other comfortable shoes in the store? A promise of an exchange is not satisfactory. If you're suspect of the store, get the guarantee of a refund in writing.

19. Next, take the shoes home and wear them for about two hours. But remember that

144

they must be kept clean—just in case! During your two hour testing wear a large pair of socks or fabric shoe bags *over* the shoes.

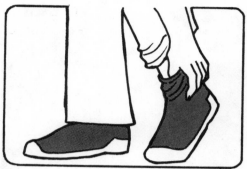

Sitting time does not count. Instead of watching television, clean out that closet you should have gotten to six months ago.

The shoes should be comfortable. Shoes should not have to be "broken in." What you actually do in "breaking in" shoes is to "break down" your feet through irritation and friction. Assuming that you must torture yourself every time you buy a new pair of shoes is an old wives' tale. The shoes may be stiff, but should not be painful!

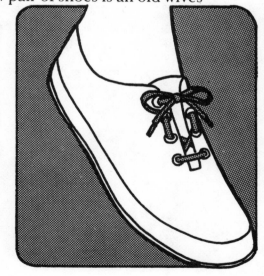

Well, all this sounds like a good deal of trouble for a pair of shoes, but remember how you've been complaining that no shoe ever fits you? And don't forget that, in spite of all this, it may well be your feet, not the shoes, that are

145

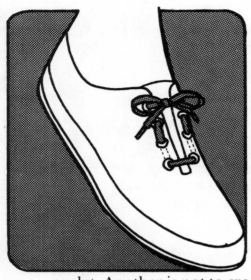

the source of your discomfort.

I have a suggestion for the man whose only shoe complaint is irritation on the top of the foot where the laces press down on a bony prominence. (A woman wearing oxfords may have the same problem.) First determine where the pressure falls. Then lace around it. One way is to cross the laces only at every other eyelet. Another is not to cross the laces until you reach the top eyelets. A multitude of ideas for lacing will come to you as you start experimenting.

In conventional shoe lacing the laces need not be pulled tightly across the top of the foot. Your shoe will stay on if only the very top crossing is snug.

If it's difficult for you to bend down to lace your

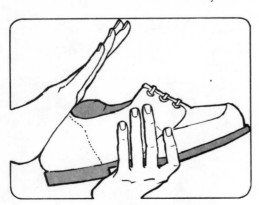

shoes, buy a pair of elasticized laces. With these you can slip into the shoe without opening the laces. If you have difficulty finding them, try one of the rehabilitation supply firms.

If there is pressure from the metal eyelets of a laced shoe, have the

146

metal removed.

If the only discomfort is caused by the stiffness of the back of the shoe, you might try "rolling" it gently with the heel of the palm of your hand. This should ease the stiffness.

Using a shoehorn will prolong the life of a shoe. Shoehorns are available in lengths up to 24 inches. If holding a shoehorn is a problem for you, there is a smooth plastic device that can be put over the back of a shoe to allow the foot to slip easily into it without a shoehorn. The one I know about is called "Insert-a-Foot Shoe Aid."

The sole of a new shoe is often so stiff that it does not bend with the foot in walking. This causes slipping at the back of the shoe. The back fit often improves if the shoe is worn long enough for the sole to flex with the foot. Test the shoes at home, *keeping them covered,* to see whether the heel problem disappears.

Sometimes the back of the shoe slips simply because the back of the shoe is too big for your foot. There are various ways to take in the back of a shoe, but except in the open-heel shoe, they are often expensive and seldom successful.

If, in shoes that you've been wearing, there is pressure on one area, as the fifth toe, try having the shoe wet lasted. Wet lasting is a shoe cobbler's term for spot stretching. Plan to leave the shoes with him for perhaps forty-eight hours. The resulting small bulge will give you greater comfort and it won't be noticeable to anyone else. If your shoe was bought from a reliable shoe man, he might do the wet lasting for you—and do a knowledgeable, responsible job.

One other word about shoes and shoe sizes. When

you are eyeing your shoes from the style critic's point of view, *don't* look down at them. Look in a mirror. No one, but no one, can possibly see your shoes from the angle you see them when you look down. The mirror sees them as others do—and they always look smaller and more stylish that way!

If you must buy shoes for a shut-in who cannot get to a shoe store, make an outline of each foot. Get from your podiatrist the name of a competent person in a reputable shoe store. Take the outlines to him. If he is of the caliber to fit a shoe this way, undoubtedly he will agree to your returning the shoes if they don't fit adequately.

If you have feet markedly different from each other in size, you'll have to buy two pairs of shoes unless you can find a shoe man who will sell you "split sizes" —one shoe from each of two pairs. Some years ago this was possible: the consumer paid a price greater than the cost of one pair of shoes, but less than the cost of two pairs. Today it is difficult to find a shoe store that will do this.

If your shoes get soaked in the rain or snow, don't— please don't—dry them near a radiator, where the heat will cause shrinkage. Stuff them with newspaper or tissue paper and put them off in a corner for a couple of days.

Shoe trees are great—for the manufacturer of the shoe trees. Why on earth should you get a pair of shoes to conform comfortably to your feet and then put shoe trees into them to eradicate the foot-fitting contours? Why not just stuff them gently with tissue paper to avoid having them crushed in your closet? If they're kept in boxes or shoe drawers, even that isn't necessary.

Have you ever wondered how shoe styles come to be? Of course, there are the commercial factors of stimulating business for the shoe industry by forcing style-conscious people to discard the shoes of last season. There are sheer utility factors such as the need for a broad-based secure shoe for hiking. There is the excellent Munson last, named after Major Edward Lyman Munson, Jr., who developed a last really shaped to a foot for use by men in the military service.

As I write this, however, I wonder how often utility is completely ignored. Think, for instance, of the absurdly high platform shoes and clogs in which women have been clomping along crowded city streets. Do you remember the game I said I play, judging the age of the person in front of me by the gait? These high platforms and clogs add a startling new dimension to my game. The wearer is ageless. It must be a robot! It can't be a human because first one foot is raised and then, with no flexibility, plopped down. Then the other is raised and—plop! it hits the pavement. Mary Ann Crenshaw, a feature writer for the *New York Times,* headed an article on these shoes, "Doctors Predict a Broken Foot." The title of the article was to the point. The falls, the injuries, the sprains and the fractures that have been caused by these shoes have been so numerous that there has been a concerted condemnation by doctors and by magazine and newspaper feature writers. Radio and television programs have highlighted the perils of these styles. Ralph Nader has made them the object of one of his investigations. And many women, as well as some men, have gone right on wearing them!

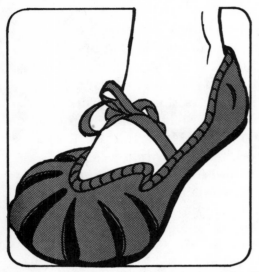

Shoe styles have sometimes come about through pathologic necessity. King Henry VIII had gout. He finally had wide shoes made to avoid pressure on his inflamed, aching feet. Actually they were soft, wide sandals with slits to prevent any toe irritation. His courtiers made these wide sandals the style of the day. The masses proceeded to outdo the courtiers. Finally the shoes were being made so wide that it was difficult for people to pass each other in the street. The situation became so acute that Henry decreed that the width of the commoners' shoes could not exceed four inches and that of the nobles' six inches.

Louis XIV is credited with introducing the high heel. Though he was very fashion conscious, he was short of stature. Wearing high-heeled shoes increased his height. Thus the high heel was born—and soon Louis XIV was surrounded by courtiers growing taller as the days went by. In that same era fashionable women began to wear high heels.

It was because of foot problems, in this case not those of royalty, that today's molded shoes came into being. Molded shoes are made to cast. There are cautions that you should keep in mind if you plan to spend the rather considerable sum charged for these shoes. Some of the firms making them knowingly, not maliciously, fit the shoes short. They reason that the backward pressure will force the toes to flex. I am not alone in believing this is harmful and can cause nail problems, as well as pressure problems, on the toes.

More often than not, molded shoes are made without a doctor's prescription or even a doctor's reference to a specific firm. These shoes are not panaceas! You should have a diagnosis of your foot problem before you have them made. You should know whether the shoes will help your condition, and whether there is any less obvious disorder that requires treatment.

The molded shoe is perhaps the most contemporary of footgear to originate because of a physical problem and to sift down to the "masses" as a shoe style. Some years ago the secretary of one of the foremost leaders in the fashion world had more than a little misgiving about confronting her employer with her new molded shoes. Finally, entering the inner sanctum, she hesitantly inquired, "Do you mind my wearing them here?"

Her employer studied the big, awkwardly contoured shoes for a moment and then asked, "Are you comfortable in them?"

"Yes, but I know that they aren't stylish and they're not right for our style reputation."

Only an established leader in the fashion world could have dismissed the matter with, "Then we'll make them stylish!"

Within a few months a Fifth Avenue shop, famous in New York for its high-styled merchandise, had an entire window display of ready-made shoes that looked exactly like molded shoes. They were, moreover, in a variety of colors. They sold quickly as the

151

"latest style." Soon patients began to ask for prescriptions for the actual molded shoes. These requests were based not on physical need, but on such considerations as, "How stylish the shoes are with sport clothes! I want the real thing, not just a copy!"

Such pseudo-molded shoes continue on the market. They are not made to cast, but are made on fairly wide lasts. They are much less expensive than the real thing, but they certainly make no allowance for specific structural abnormalities of the feet.

Most of us wear shoes long enough to need some shoe repairs. Certainly heels should not be permitted to be run down. Not only is your appearance less than neat and affluent, but your gait is thrown out of kilter. Frequently I have found the answer to a patient's fatigue or leg pain in simply advising him to have new lifts. As I have said, rubber lifts are more shock absorbing and more slip-proof than lifts made of other materials.

I keep harking back to warnings about promised cure-alls and I include cure-all advice from your shoe cobbler. Often he will advise metal heel guards to avoid running down the heels. A mail order house advertises such guards:

> No More Shoddy Run-Down Heels! . . . last for months and attach easily to rubber or leather. Set includes complete materials for 3 pairs of heels. Cut repair costs for the whole family! Always put them on your new shoes.

And all this for only one dollar! Whether you are a do-it-yourselfer or a shoe cobbler's customer, avoid these guards. They simply compound your foot problem and thus may eventually demand more of your pocketbook. Nor should you attach them at the front tip of the shoe. If you've already bought them and now wonder what to do with them, you might try adding them as decorations to your youngster's building blocks—or just throw them out!

Your shoe cobbler may try to be helpful by suggesting wedging the shoe at areas of wear. Thank him for his interest. And don't have it done. His intentions are good; the results for your feet are almost always bad. Wedging should be done only on prescription.

Another version of panacea shoe wedging comes from a mail order house. Again there is no inkling of the damage that you can do by increasing the faults of your gait.

> Stop Uneven Heel Wear! If you wear down the outside edge of shoe heels, your problem may be rotating ankles. Now, rubber heel cushions help balance every step, so shoes look new longer! If you wear down inside edge, switch cushions to opposite shoes! Order by shoe size.

Hopefully you don't wear shoes until they need resoling. Adlai Stevenson's famous hole in the sole of his shoe may have caused less of a problem for him than resoling would have. Too often the process of resoling makes the shoes too snug.

Selecting hosiery is as important as selecting shoes. Most hosiery today is made with some nylon and is of the stretch type—one size meets the requirements of a range of sizes. Women often find the selection of panty hose an expensive trial and error process. If a one-size-fits-all type of panty hose is not available, knowing your stocking size may be helpful.

The following table, compiled by the Podiatry

Society of the State of New York, *approximates* the hosiery sizes of men and women in relationship to shoe sizes:

Ladies'		Men's	
Shoe	Hose	Shoe	Hose
2½–3½	8½	5½–6	9½
4 –4½	9	6½–7	10
5 –5½	9½	7½–8	10½
6 –6½	10	8½–9	11
7 –7½	10½	9½–10	11½
8 up	11	10½–11	12
		11½–12	13

Hopefully yours is not the situation of a patient who consulted me many years ago. He was eight feet six inches tall and wore a size 21 shoe. His socks were hand knitted.

Lisle socks, cotton socks and wool socks are the most absorbent and consequently the most comfortable. Nylons are not absorbent and they aggravate excessive perspiration. (Some nylon hosiery is made with cotton feet, but it may be difficult to find.) It is

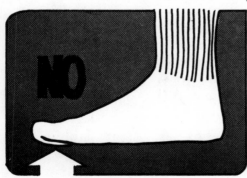

true, of course, that hosiery of nylon fits better than that of other materials. If you wear hosiery that is not nylon, avoid tucking the toe area under your foot. This inevitably interferes with normal flexion of your toes.

I have already pointed out that support hosiery is a triumph in advertising, but not a miracle in treatment. The very quality that makes it supportive on the leg becomes a constricting factor on the foot. This constriction can aggravate nail problems, soft corns and other foot lesions. If you need supportive hosiery for a leg condition such as varicose veins, have toeless surgical stockings made to wear under your street hosiery. One can also buy ready-made surgical stockings at a pharmacy.

Current styles in women's boots have much to recommend them—and much to make one cautious about them. A major problem is the leg fit. A woman with a heavy leg may have great difficulty finding a boot that is not too snug. Excessive boot constriction at the leg is thought to be a cause of circulatory problems such as phlebitis.

Some high styled boots have heels that are too high for secure walking on icy surfaces. Style can be combined with a moderate heel, an adequately roomy leg fit and a wide base, making for the ideal cold weather footgear. Any modification or arch supports that have been prescribed can, moreover, be worn in a boot that fits properly.

I think back to the time when we wore heavy boots over shoes. The boot of today is far superior—for outdoor use. In my opinion, boots should not be worn a full day indoors. At best they are certainly more constricting and less flexible than shoes.

Chapter 12

Your Feet Are on the Job, Too!

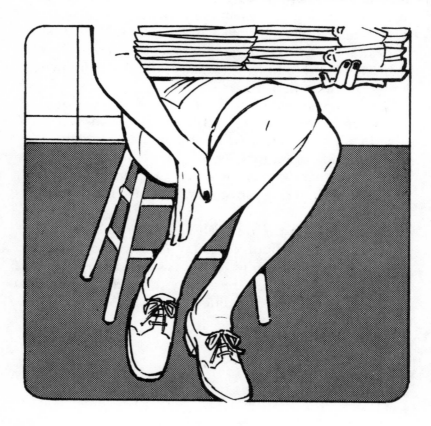

A massive chunk of our lives is spent on the job—be it that of the salesman, the waitress, the dentist, the housewife, the policeman, the farmer or any other of a multitude of occupations.

Perhaps you're one of the vast number of people who have suffered—and may still be suffering—from an accident or disease that is occupation-related. Dr. P. Lewin states in his text, *The Foot and Ankle:*

> The chief causes of industrial disabilities are sprains, strains, ruptures, dislocations and diseases occurring in the foot and ankle. Trauma is much more frequently responsible than disease.

Because of the tremendous expense to industry in absenteeism, lowered efficiency and compensation costs resulting from foot problems, more and more large business concerns have added podiatrists to their medical staffs. Many smaller firms have arranged for periodic visits of their personnel to the offices of podiatrists.

157

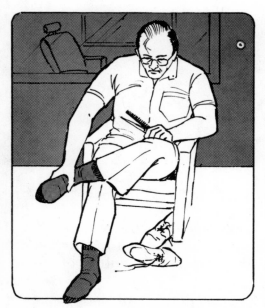

Certain disabilities are peculiar to certain occupations. A good example is the foot strain of which many waitresses and barbers complain. These people spend most of their working day on their feet, often in less than optimum shoes. The waitress has the additional disadvantage of carrying heavy trays. The barber spends much of his time standing in one place. Standing is more difficult than walking. The complaint of people in such occupations generally is, "My feet hurt all over. I'm dead tired at the end of the day."

Many are the salespeople, the checkout clerks, the household workers, the mechanics—and the executives—who would be more successful in their person-to-person relationships were they not battling against the constant awareness of foot pain. One of my patients always remarks at the end of his periodic treatments, "Today I'll be good to my customers."

Frequently, however, foot problems do not truly result from the demands of the job. They existed, perhaps with severe symptoms, before that specific occupation was undertaken. If, for instance, you have poor foot posture and poor gait, and then get a job as a butcher or an elevator operator, the constant standing will obviously aggravate the condition, leading possibly to extreme fatigue, lower back discomfort, and leg and foot pains.

The cost in comfort and in efficiency is great, but the cost in safety might be far more catastrophic. The Industrial Commission of Ohio cites the case of a man whose bunion was so painful that he had to take his weight off his foot. To do this he supported himself by resting his elbow on the edge of his whirling machine. Less alert than he might have been had he had no pain, he miscalculated by a few inches—and his elbow was caught in the machine.

Timely professional foot care could have prevented this accident.

There is a correlation between certain hazards and certain occupations.

Repeated small injuries may cause enough damage to be equal to or greater than the damage of one massive injury. Ballet dancers are often heir to such conditions. The person constantly on a ladder, such as the painter or the displayman, subjects his feet to constant small injuries. Although these people most often complain of pain at the ball of the foot, frequently the pain is less readily localized. "My feet hurt all over!" The delivery man, jumping down from a truck many times a day, may develop a stress fracture.

Workers in slippery areas must be cautioned again and again against falling. Having gotten along day after day without mishap, they become careless—until suddenly down they go. Fractures of any part of the body may result, but very often it is the hip, leg or ankle that is broken.

Metal workers, such as foundrymen, often burn

their feet and legs in pouring hot metal. People working with chemicals frequently drop substances on their feet or legs causing burns and ulcerations.

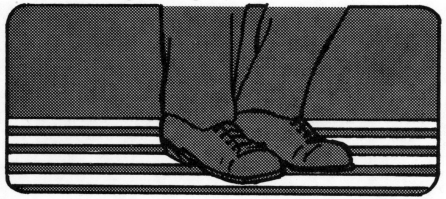

Those who are constantly in moist, warm areas may develop fungous infections of the feet. Bartenders, dishwashers, laundresses, bathhouse attendants, workers in greenhouses and hairdressers are exposed to this type of environment. Where it is at all feasible, it is certainly desirable to stand on a wide slatted surface that will at least permit drainage.

Each occupation has its own built-in hazards and you learn quickly—hopefully just conversationally—what are those in your work.

What can you do about it? You can assume that you're not immune, and that those who take precautions aren't sissies! Fortunately, various industries make safety shoes mandatory. Whether or not you wear safety shoes, be sure your shoes fit comfortably. You need the security of comfort when you are on your feet. Have treatment for any discomfort with which you've come to the job and continue treatment to maintain your comfort. Many a fracture might have been avoided if the victim had been more sure-footed!

160

And don't feel smug in your sense of security if you're a housewife! The danger of accidents in your home is tremendous, the more because there's no boss to enforce safety rules. Wrinkled carpets, throw rugs, too softly lit stairways, frayed carpeting on stairs, highly polished floors—all are traps with no danger signs.

Standing on boxes or chairs or half-opened ladders invites disaster. Getting out of bed in the dark and stumbling half-asleep into a piece of furniture is the usual story of a fracture of a toe, frequently the fifth toe. This happens so often that the term "bedroom fracture" is commonly used.

A less dramatic danger than a fracture exists in the use of kitchen and bathroom carpeting, which is a veritable haven for various organisms and fungi. Remember that fungous infections can readily be spread from one person to another, particularly on moist, porous surfaces.

Particles of skin of a person with a fungous infection become lodged in the carpeting and then contaminate the next barefoot member of the household.

Research has shown that kitchen and bathroom carpeting cannot be cleaned as thoroughly as a nonporous surface such as vinyl.

Chapter **13**
What's Your Sport?

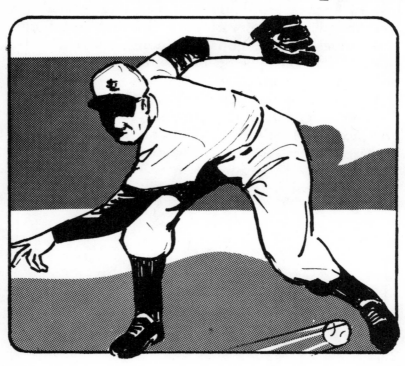

Today, just about everyone does have a sport—and those who can't lay claim to even one such activity are almost apologetic.

The day is gone when, after graduation from school, one's physical activity was limited to the job, a softball game at the annual family picnic, and an occasional evening on the dance floor.

Today, even dancing is an athletic feat in itself. Now, along with jogger's ankle, tennis toe, and runner's knee, we have disco foot.

And this participation in sports is all for the good. We stay younger and healthier when we use our bodies. But we must recognize the need for certain precautions.

Our feet, perhaps more than any other part of the body, take the brunt of use—and overuse—in this current spurt of sports. In running, for instance, the additional force bearing down on your feet and legs may be two, three, or even four times your body weight. Hal Higdon, writing in *Runner's World* (April 1978), points out that a 130-pound person, in running, might be exerting 400 pounds of pressure on his or her legs. "Multiply that by 5,000 steps taken during a typical hour's run, and you get tremendous forces applied on the lower extremities of the body."

Any disability resulting either from overuse or injury to your feet or legs affects the rest of your body and, at the least, interferes with your performance—or, even worse, eliminates you permanently from your sport.

A sad illustration of this was within the career of Dizzy Dean, who signed his first contract to play baseball in 1929.

"As a ballplayer, Dean was a natural phenomenon, like the Grand Canyon or the Great Barrier Reef," according to a lengthy *New York Times* article that appeared when he died on July 17, 1974.

Things started to unwind in 1937, when Dean was struck on the left foot by a line drive while pitching in the All-Star Game in Washington. He suffered a fractured toe, but suffered more permanently when he tried to pitch despite the handicap, subsequently ruining his right arm.

The caption below a picture read, "Dizzy Dean pitching in 1937, the year his career was cut short when he changed delivery because of a toe injury."

Whether your sport is jogging or roller-skating or backpacking or cross-country skiing or tennis or adventure running or just about any other activity beyond television dozing, listen to the experts. It is no mere coincidence that in each area you'll be told:

1. Before you start, make sure your body is in good condition.
2. Buy proper equipment for your sport.
3. Do warm-up exercises.

164

4. Learn proper technique.

5. Don't play through or run through pain.

Let's discuss these precautions.

1. Before you start, make sure your body is in good condition. "We've had a motto around the office for some years now which states that you should get in shape to play tennis, not play tennis to get in shape." I am quoting the editor of *Tennis* magazine, Shepherd Campbell.

If, indeed, we delete the word *tennis,* we might well substitute the name of any other sport—skiing, squash, sprinting, jogging, golf, or what have you.

Have your physician examine you. This should be a must for everyone initially embarking on any sports activity, with double emphasis on the sedentary person and the person over fifty.

Dr. Richard O. Schuster, a New York podiatrist of national repute, who has been called the guru of runners, states that "because certain activities such as running result in unusual stress on the foot, athletes have unique podiatric problems. Often a minor structural weakness

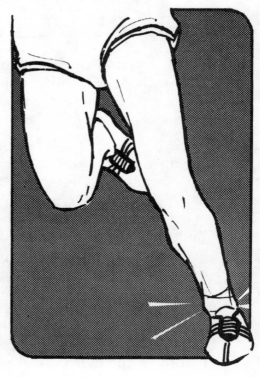

165

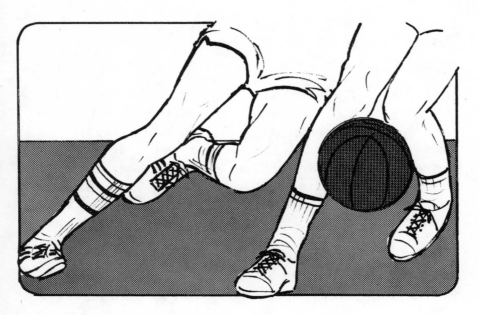

which would be asymptomatic in the average person causes discomfort when subjected to vigorous athletic activities. Repeated insult despite pain aggravates the problem."

Dr. Schuster lends emphasis to my consistent urging that you seek a diagnosis and treatment for any discomfort or disability. "Repeated insult despite pain aggravates the problem."

Dr. Paul Taylor, team podiatrist for the Washington Bullets of the National Basketball Association, estimates that 75 percent of injuries occur to the knees, ankles, and feet. In speaking of basketball players, in the *Journal of the American Podiatry Association,* March 1974, he stressed a fundamental point: "Foot problems in basketball are really problems common to all of us, but due to the constant running and jumping that the game demands, they become more serious."

166

With less-than-optimum health you more quickly reach a dangerous degree of fatigue. With fatigue, judgement becomes less accurate, carelessness more prevalent—and you may well be headed for disaster.

The statistics of the United States Consumer Product Safety Commission reflecting injuries treated in hospital emergency rooms, from January 1, 1978 to December 31, 1978, reveal that 36,983 occurred during gymnastics and the use of associated equipment, and, of these, 15,960 involved the lower extremities. Of the 48,983 injuries resulting from tennis, badminton, and squash, 24,802 involved the lower extremities. The total figure for dancing injuries treated in hospital emergency rooms was 2,714, with 1,956 referable to the lower extremities.

The figures emphasize two factors:

You need the alertness that comes of good overall health, including the stability, coordination, and surefootedness of an optimally aligned body resting on a base of properly functioning feet.

You need proper equipment.

2. Buy proper equipment for your sport. Tennis shoes are not adequate for jogging. The jogging shoe has a wedged heel that minimizes pull on the muscles and tendons at the back of your leg.

Brand names mean far less than does a comfortable, well-fitted shoe, whether it be a running shoe or a tennis sneaker. When the shoe is fitted, wear the hosiery—one or two pairs—that you plan to wear with the shoe.

Sizes may differ considerably from those of your

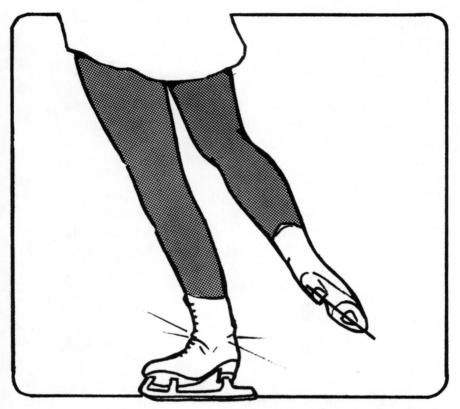

street shoes. Women often find that men's sneakers or running shoes fit better than those designed specifically for women.

Again there is the problem that we discussed before—the fact that all shoes are sold in pairs, though no one of us has a *pair* of feet. Since, even though you may have a significant difference in size, you can't buy a right sneaker or running shoe for your right foot and a left one for your left foot unless you go to the expense of two pairs of shoes, at least fit your larger foot properly, and attempt a filler in the shoe of the smaller foot.

168

Don't accept the euphoric claims of manufacturers that the shoe has a built-in "arch support." If your feet need support, you need the advice of a podiatrist or an orthopedist.

Safety precaution dictates knowing where you are going to use your equipment. Peter Wood, in *The Book of Squash* (Van Nostrand Reinhold, New York, 1972), states, "As for sneakers, comfort is the prime consideration. If the courts you are playing on have been painted properly . . . that is, if the right amount of pumice has been added to the paint on the floor . . . slipping should be no problem. If, however, the floors are slippery, sneakers with a deck-gripping tread are preferable to those with a smooth rubber sole."

Roller skaters find greater safety in boot skates, with the boot attached to the skate plate and wheels, than in the older type of skate that clamped onto the shoe.

For backpacking on most trails a medium-weight boot is recommended. Lee Schreiber in *Backpacking* (Stein and Day, New York, 1978) a book written with the editors of *Backpacking Journal,* warns, "Sure, it's entirely possible to hike in sneakers or running shoes or sandals. But the end of such a day would bring uncomfortable results: sore, aching, hot feet with a mass of bad blisters. Added to this will be overtired legs and a generally fatigued body because of the extra exertion necessary to make up for the footwear problems. . . . Remember these results when you're having second thoughts about spending . . . [the money] for a pair of good, well-fitted hiking boots."

While buying desirable footgear may be expensive, renting it may be more expensive—in performance and pain and possibly even money.

When Lisa, a sixteen-year-old patient of mine, left for a month's hiking vacation, she was bubbling with delight in her newly found foot comfort and with enthusiasm for her contemplated trip. She disregarded my misgivings about renting hiking boots, "because the people who run this trip know exactly what we need!"

The day after Lisa's return home her mother called for an appointment for her daughter "as soon as you possibly can see her."

Vacations are precious and I was sad as Lisa described to me the pain that she had experienced constantly in the rented boots—and the three days that she had been forced to stay at the base while the others went ahead—because she had to stay off her feet.

"I guess, Dr. Roberts, I should have bought hiking boots and had you adjust them as you wanted to," she lamented. If she had, she probably would have had a whopping vacation.

I must tell you about another patient who for many years subjected herself to that destructive philosophy of "I can't."

Ruth is thirty-two now, and a new joy has come to her. When she first consulted me, she told me that John, her fiance, was an avid skater.

"Do you enjoy ice skating?" I asked.

"No! I can't skate," she admitted sadly.

Looking at her neglected feet, I could readily understand this.

"Haven't you tried?"

Yes, she had—even when she was younger, but,

"My ankles have always been weak and the shoes always hurt me." Ruth had never tried to find out the reason for the weakness of her ankles—and she had never owned a pair of ice skates. She had always rented skates. She would buy a pair, she reasoned, when she was good enough to enjoy skating.

Now, because of John, ice skating had become really important to her.

I demonstrated that her ankles were weak because her feet were not in the correct position and, therefore, were not supporting her ankles.

We started treatment, after having agreed that she would buy—not rent—skates.

About ten weeks later Ruth bought her shoes and had the skates attached. I modified the inside of the shoes to keep her feet and ankles in the optimal position. Now, five years later, Ruth thoroughly enjoys skating with John—and each Christmas she sends me a card with a picture of a skating rink on it.

I have spoken primarily of shoes, though, indeed, necessary safety equipment may include much in addition to shoes. In roller skating, for instance, knee pads, elbow pads, and gloves may save you from serious injury.

It is wise to consult with a pro in the sport in which you are a beginner and to read some of the books that are proliferating on almost every sport.

3. Do warm-up exercises. You'll be hard put to find a currently written book or article about any sport that doesn't at least comment on the necessity for warm-up exercises each time before you start.

And don't for one minute think that disco dancing

is not included. Dr. Joseph C. D'Amico, chairman of
the Division of Orthopedic Sciences at the New York
College of Podiatric Medicine, urges "that participants treat disco dancing like an athletic endeavor—
which it is—and establish a routine of warm-up exercises before going out onto the dance floor."

Well, it *is* different from a Viennese waltz!

Warm-up exercises are of two types, those for
strengthening muscle and those for stretching muscle.

Obviously, the salient muscles to be strengthened
vary from sport to sport. However, I remind you again
and again that the body is a total unit; what happens
to one part of the body affects other parts of the body
and optimum function of any kind is dependent on
total body coordination. Thus, while weight lifting
may demand more of the upper body, woe unto you
if your feet or legs collapse when you are under a
150-pound barbell.

Books written about your specific sport interest invariably list strengthening and stretching exercises designed for that sport.

Bob Anderson, author and publisher of the book
Stretching (Anderson Press, California, 1975), general-
izes about stretching exercises. "The long, sustained
stretch . . . is a far superior method of stretching
the musculature and surrounding connective tissue
than the bouncing . . . stretch."

In speaking of the duration of stretching, he advises,
"Get used to feeling an 'easy' stretch, a stretch that
feels good, for fifteen to thirty seconds . . . the longer
you hold an 'easy' stretch, the less you will feel the
stretch tension."

He warns, "You should not stretch to the point
of pain. This is not the way to get the maximum bene-

fit from stretching. Stretching *as far as you can* is over-stretching. . . ." As important as the warm-up before your sport activity is the cool-down after it.

Nina Kuscsik in the September 1979 *Runner* magazine describes the cool-down as "actually the warm-up process in reverse." And, indeed, it is, since athletes should finish their activity with stretching exercises.

I certainly can't vouch for the whole world of athletes, but, being an early riser myself, I have seen, even before sunrise, stretching exercises being meticulously performed by men and women athletes in the parks and on the streets from New York City to Peking. The very universality of it attests to the good that is derived.

4. Learn proper technique. Let me tell you of a man who is alert enough to know when his technique is failing him.

He isn't an athlete. He had no foot pain. When first he came to my office, though, he was tremendously distressed.

He is a professional violinist, a man of some repute. For a time he had sensed that his violin playing was below his optimum. Now he felt there was a conspicuous change. It was not that he was playing incorrect notes or that his timing was poor. His music simply no longer had the vibrancy it once possessed.

Then, shortly before his visit to me, he had read a book, *The Art of Violin Playing* (Fisher, New York, 1956), by Carl Flesch. "Even the simplest movements of the arms can be carried out properly only when the position of the legs is correspondingly correct . . . it is necessary to stand firmly on both feet."

173

This was his reason for consulting me. He did, indeed, have faulty foot posture. As treatment progressed, his playing improved.

Perhaps I was as happy as he when he came in beaming, "I'm back to myself again."

And certainly technique in any sport is specific to that sport, but without proper foot function, you may strike a sour note.

5. Don't play through or run through pain. Pain is a signal. Pain is to be respected. We should be thankful for it.

By the time you experience pain you're beginning to be in trouble. Continuing with the activity that's causing you pain begs for body damage. Perhaps you've already "pulled a muscle" or developed an inflammation of a tendon.

Isn't it pretty obvious that continuing to put stress on these areas will aggravate the problem—and very likely keep you out of your sport over a prolonged period?

These five important precautions are so basic to athletic participation that they merit being repeated.

1. Before you start, make sure your body is in good condition.
2. Buy proper equipment for your sport.
3. Do warm-up exercises.
4. Learn proper technique.
5. Don't play through or run through pain.

Each sport, of course, has its own requirements. The roller skating we did as youngsters is different

174

in many respects from the roller skating that is gaining so many adult devotees that currently 300,000 pairs of skates a month are being sold, with sales 50 percent behind demand.

Skate wheels used to be made of steel. Today they are made of polyurethane, which permits greater speed than was possible on the steel wheels.

The greater speed brings with it greater threats to safety. In the first nine months of 1978, 70,000 patients with roller-skating injuries were treated in hospital emergency rooms. Of these, 20,000 had ankle sprains or strains, and 25,000 had injuries to the upper extremities.

For this reason, skaters are urged to learn how to wrap their arms around themselves and roll when they fall. I've mentioned the knee pads, elbow pads, and gloves that are part of the recommended equipment. Wrist guards and even padded shorts are also advised.

In *Anybody's Roller Skating Book* (Bantam, New York, 1979), Tom Cuthbertson gives many suggestions for the beginner. Among them is, "Work at developing strong ankles so that you can coast easily . . . and get speed from neat strokes that have no extra motion."

But how do you develop strong ankles? Let's remember that your ankles can't be strong if your feet, which are the foundation below them, are out of line. You can exercise from now until doomsday, but, if, with each step you come down on the wrong parts of your feet, your ankles will be wobbly and insecure.

Try putting one box on top of another. Then tilt the bottom box. Does the top one stay in its original place?

If your ankles are weak, nine chances out of ten

your podiatrist will find a faulty functioning of your feet, not a weakness inherent in your ankles.

Dr. John Pagliano, president of the American Academy of Podiatric Sports Medicine, stresses that "excellent-fitting skate boots and proper conditioning are two of the most important warnings we can give to the neophyte skater. . . . The boot should fit snugly . . . and provide enough room for toe swelling, which is brought on by the excess perspiration the sport generates."

Cotton socks absorb perspiration much better than synthetics do.

The boot, while it should be snug, should certainly be comfortable from the outset, with no need for "breaking in."

If you need a modification or a mould in the boot to maintain your foot and ankle position, be sure that the boot is fitted to allow the necessary space.

Tennis has gained an amazing popularity in recent years. Players vie for time on open courts and in "bubbles." Entire stores are devoted to equipment and apparel for that one sport.

Tennis, like any other sport, requires warm-up exercises, and tennis, like any other sport, has its own contingencies. The type of court is a factor. Courts of clay and grass are the easiest for your feet.

Tennis toe is a hemorrhaging that occurs at the tip of your toe or under your toenail. It happens because: (1) your tennis shoe is too short; or (2) because your tennis shoe has so much traction that your foot, in sudden stops, is jammed against the front of the shoe; or (3) because your feet are not functioning properly and consequently are sliding forward in your shoes.

176

The area becomes discolored, and painful, and it often throbs. Your podiatrist should be consulted, not only to treat the painful area, but also to determine whether the problem is inherent in your foot posture. Don't count on the construction of your tennis shoe to hold your foot properly!

Tennis and other racquet sports also make great demands on the back of the leg. Frequently there are injuries to the leg muscles or to the Achilles tendon, which is the heavy tendon that you can feel at the lower part of the back of the leg. There may be an inflammation of the area, Achilles tendinitis, or even a rupture, or tearing, of part of the tendon. These problems, too, can generally be avoided by proper warm-up and by proper foot function.

These precautions will also help to avoid pain in your heels and in the bottom of your feet.

Disco foot is the latest addition to our expository list of sport ailments. Dr. D'Amico describes disco foot as "a painful combination of sprains, fractures, minor bursitis, and excessive fatigue."

Discotheque dancing is certainly akin to other athletic endeavors, with the additional impediment for women of outrageously high stiletto heels that are a threat when walking in the street, let alone stomping and twisting on a slippery dance floor in a relatively small area of activity.

Last June I was invited to a reception for a graduate of a professional school. The music was constant and all that the discotheque dancer could want.

Among the guests was a patient of mine, a twenty-five-year-old professional dancer. I had been strapping her foot and ankle for several weeks. She still had on her left foot, reaching up to the lower third of her leg, the strapping that I had applied two days before.

As I watched her dance, I smiled at the obvious superiority of her skill and grace. She truly stood out in the crowd.

And I got to thinking to myself, "Why am I still treating Marcey? She seems great!"

Three dances later I watched her leave the floor. She was beginning to limp. Two dances after that she left the floor more slowly and with an obviously worsening limp.

"Indeed," I thought, "I'll be strapping her forever—and never with any lasting results!"

Drs. J. Gorman, B. Helfand, and R. Mazer, all Pennsylvania podiatrists, write of the disco injuries that are, more commonly than not, the result of overuse. Frequently continuing pain develops in the ball of the foot and in the legs. Fatigue and lower back pain are often experienced. At the extreme, stress fractures occur from the constant overuse of the feet—particularly if the feet are not in prime condition. Since many of the participants in discotheque dancing are young people who dress in high fashion and who fear being advised to change their shoe styles, they don't seek professional advice as soon as they should—at the first sign of pain or evidently excessive fatigue.

Much can be done, even within the framework of "fashion" shoes, to help the disco dancer.

To go to the extreme opposite from stiletto heels, let's talk about skiing.

Skiing injuries are enjoyed by no one except the

178

cartoonist. It is well accepted that most skiing accidents—as well as accidents in other sports—occur when one of our five basic rules is defied. Fatigue is often responsible for accidents—the tired skier's attitude of "just once more." That "once more" is the skier's undoing.

Many improvements have been made in skis and in boots. Skis are shorter; boots cause fewer leg fractures.

But the improvement in the basic factory construction of boots may not be adequate to meet your own, individual foot requirements. Your orthopedist or your podiatrist should examine you and prescribe any mould or modification that, by improving your body coordination and minimizing your fatigue, will add to your safety.

Just as in the early hours of the morning, I see men and women doing their stretching exercises, so I see men and women of varying ages jogging or running. Some almost glide with ease and pleasure; some seem so desperate with tension and strain that I fear for their well-being. Some clomp along with such a lack of grace that I honestly have been tempted—but I haven't done it—to stop them to explain that with good foot balance they could at least stop clomping and start jogging!

Jogging is the term generally used when one's speed is slower than nine minutes a mile. Completing a mile in less than nine minutes is considered running.

Jogging actually consists of walking and running alternately. The American Podiatry Association recommends the following timetable for the beginning jogger.

(1–6 weeks)

Warm up with walking and stretching movement.

Jog 55 yards, walk 55 yards (four times).
Jog 110 yards, walk 110 yards (four times).
Jog 55 yards, walk 55 yards (four times).

Pace 110 yards in about forty-five seconds.

(6–12 weeks)

Increase jogging and reduce walking.
Pace 110 yards in thirty to thirty-seven seconds.

(12–24 weeks)

Jog a nine-minute mile.

(30+ weeks)

The second workout each week, add variety—
continuous jogging, or running and walking alternately at a slow varying pace for distances up
to two miles.

Both joggers and runners sometimes set for themselves unrealistic—or at least unhealthy—goals either
in time or distance or both. I was in charge of one
of the medical stations in Central Park during the
New York Marathon in 1978. On the 26-mile run,
this station was at 24.6 miles.

When Bill Rodgers, ahead of the others, came by
at an easy, steady pace, he was unruffled, despite the
heat of the day. He looked as though he might just
have run around the block—and leisurely, at that.

Then, for the next two hours or so, came men and
women of various ages, various forms, various speeds,
and various intensities. Some were keeping a steady

pace, grateful for a cup of water either to drink or to douse over their heads; some were panting so badly that I was relieved that they dropped out at our station for a few minutes. All of them were able to resume running.

Then late, late—almost three hours after Bill Rodgers had gone by—came some straining stragglers whose stoicism I admired more than their wisdom. I wonder how their bodies fared the next several days!

The very last man I saw had reached the finish line at 26 miles and had then started walking back because he lived in the area of our station at 90th Street off Fifth Avenue. When I saw him, he was bare-footed and dragging himself toward me just as I was about to leave.

His feet were completely covered with huge blood blisters. Some had already broken and the blood was oozing out as he stumbled along the dirty road. He had, indeed, reached the finish line—and he had done it in proper running shoes—and no socks, as is the preference of some runners.

For this man, though he lived close by, the only possible answer was the ambulance that I called to take him to a hospital.

Dr. Schuster has said that all runners hurt sooner or later, and that most injuries start after 25 miles. His preference is for afternoon running. In the September 1979 *Runner* magazine he commented, "Most people get hurt in the morning. They're so damn anxious to get on with the day that they don't want to take the time to warm up and stretch those muscles. They're also groggy that early in the day."

Runners, being almost as addicted to runners' reading as to running itself, know a good deal about what

181

the contingencies are, where their bodies are most likely to develop trouble. Unfortunately they are not always proficient at differential diagnosis or at therapy. Consequently they sometimes misdiagnose their own problems and too often decide that an "orthotic" will be the magic therapy that will promptly—in fact, tomorrow—get them back to running. Of course, more often than not, they don't stop running even when their bodies do indeed ache.

There are various conditions that may beset the runner—and the orthotic is not always the answer, and certainly not always the immediate answer or the full answer.

Some of the problems that do arise are:

Achilles Tendinitis, an inflammation in the area of the large tendon at the back of the lower leg.

Blisters, which may come from poorly fitting shoes, from faulty foot function, from not wearing properly fitting socks, or from wearing no socks. Alas! My poor marathon runner with his blisters!

Knee Problems, which frequently derive from faulty foot function. Knee problems have always haunted athletes. Too often injections, or, even more radical, surgery was prescribed. Too often the result was an athlete's forfeiting his sport for life.

Today the initial advice for a knee problem is: "Have your feet examined." Dr. George Sheehan, the well-known cardiologist and marathon runner, is the medical editor of *Runner's World*. Consistently he has answered questions about knee problems with advice about foot stability.

Dr. Schuster attaches great importance to differences in leg lengths as a cause of foot imbalance with resulting knee conditions. Again, you must remember that, while one quarter of an inch difference may have no impact on the life of a nonathlete, the additional stress of an activity such as running may well cause a knee problem.

Morton's toe, an impingement on a nerve in the foot.

Pain Under the Heel, sometimes from a heel spur, sometimes from faulty foot function.

Runner's Toe, a blood blister at the tip of the toe or under the nail. This results from the toe hitting against the front of the shoe.

Shin Splints, strain or fatigue of the muscles of the leg, often caused by overuse and foot imbalance.

Stress Fractures, which come from banging down constantly on a bone as a result of faulty foot function.

I do admit that the phrase "faulty foot function" creeps into this book again and again, but it is the culprit for so much that interferes with our well-being and our ease in activity! And generally it responds so readily to treatment that it's just about equally culpable to accept the disability with no attempt to be helped!

183

Another type of running that is coming more and more to the fore is Adventure Running, which has been described by Jerry Schad in the February/March 1979 issue of *Mariah/Outside* as a "sport ideal for anyone who likes to combine an outdoor experience with strenuous exercise."

Adventure Running is running alone or with just a few other participants. Mr. Schad explains ". . . nor is it necessarily confined to the Grand Canyon or other spectacular parklands. Adventure running courses may be as close to home as an old logging road, forest path, firebreak, or isolated beach just outside of town. The only requirements are that they must be long or difficult enough to present a personal challenge, and that their setting be somewhat unusual—preferably wilderness or semiwildland."

Jay Longacre, tired of marathons, has run in a variety of interesting, challenging places including the Grand Canyon, the Seychelles, and the Himalayas.

Training is specialized for this kind of running. Distance is more important than speed. Running on all sorts of terrain, some of it with perhaps unpredictable hazards, is essential. And you had better have good foot stability for some of those areas.

If you're the adventurous kind of person who can enjoy new places and new sights while you're running and still show care along all kinds of terrain, perhaps this may be the sport for you. Training may be even more intensive than that for the usual mode of running. Shoe recommendations depend on the type of terrain and the season of the year.

Well, perhaps sometime you'll want to investigate adventure running.

Another great way to see the sights out there while

you're doing much to maintain a healthy body is to hike or backpack. Lee Schreiber, author of *Backpacking*, in writing of boots, makes a statement that is fundamental, although writers seem never to mention it. "While mail-order fitting is possible, the types of boot lasts used vary widely, making fitting difficult. *Thus, no boots should be mail ordered unless there is a firm return policy should the boots not fit correctly.*"

There is a warning against hiking shoes that are either too light or too heavy. "For most trail use with moderate-weight pack, a medium boot, in a range of three to four and a half pounds, is more than ample. Heavier boots will only punish you, while light shoes will do far too little to protect and support your feet when you're toting a heavy pack over rocky and rough trails."

The suggestions for the fitting of the boot are those that I have been making to you—the toe one half to three quarters of an inch beyond your longest toe, the width across the widest part of your foot not binding, but not excessively wide.

Added to your own weight is the weight of your backpack. Add to that the hazards of uneven terrain, together with the probable onset of fatigue going up and down hills, and you need little convincing that once again the importance of good foot function is paramount, not only for stability, but for minimal knee jarring.

Physical conditioning programs for backpacking might involve any of several sports such as volleyball, tennis, badminton, cycling, or swimming. Include walking briskly, first along a varied course equivalent in distance to six or seven miles. Then do the same course with a light backpack, gradually increasing the weight.

But, whether or not you're interested in hiking or backpacking, walking—just walking—is, in itself, a splendid exercise. It requires no team or opponent, no expense for equipment beyond the proper care of your feet and shoes that you probably should be wearing for your everyday use anyway, no driving out to a special area, no large chunks of your time, no showers after your exercise.

Walking, even if you can't find time for other sports, can be worked into your daily schedule in a multitude of ways.

Rain or shine, I get off my bus in the morning at a stop that gives me about a twenty-minute walk to my office. Five days a week I do this. On week-ends I miss it enough that I think up destinations just to be able to walk.

I am always dismayed when I am with someone, usually a woman, who says, "Please, please, can't we take a bus or a cab? I never walk more than a block or so."

Generally, after one glance at her shoes and at the inward throw of her ankles, the reason is clear. Yes, I always agree—because I am sorry for her. If only she had had proper care for her feet and had worn attractive, but adequate, shoes, she could have had the companionable activity of walking with the good feeling that comes of getting the body "turning over."

City folk are more fortunate than suburbanites in the fact that they walk more. Suburbanites always have the car just outside the door. Getting a container of milk means driving down to the supermarket. City folk seldom have a car in front of the door, and certainly don't fetch it from a garage or move it from a prized parking space in the street just to go for a container of milk. They walk!

186

It is not unusual for a woman who has recently moved to the city after years of living in the suburbs to make her first appointment with a podiatrist. The appointment is generally made with a good degree of urgency.

Mrs. Mills, newly arrived in New York from Larchmont, a suburb, had that same urgency in her voice when she called my office for an appointment one day last May. The history she gave me was typical.

"I never had trouble with my feet until I moved here from Larchmont last October. I'm very concerned. There are so many things here to see each day, so many places to go—and I can't go!"

Mrs. Mills, an attractive, well-dressed woman, is forty-eight years old. For twenty-five years she lived in Larchmont, keeping house and caring for her husband, her two sons, and her daughter. Now she and her husband had moved to the city.

In Larchmont she drove rather than walked. In Larchmont she wore sneakers or other casual shoes with slacks for most of her daytime chores. Now, whenever she left home she felt a need to wear, if not dressy, at least less casual, footgear. Now everywhere she went she was surrounded by crowds, with little chance to maintain a steady, easy pace.

And what was happening? All the potential problems Mrs. Mills had been harboring for years now came to the fore. It was just as much the overuse syndrome as if the symptoms had come with playing tennis or jogging.

Ruth Rudner, author of *Off and Walking* (Holt, Rinehart and Winston, New York, 1977), points out in an article in *Self,* April 1979, that "to lose one pound of fat you must use up the approximately 3,500 calories that make up that pound. The American Medical

Association says you can do just that by walking briskly one mile a day beyond what you ordinarily walk, for thirty-six days, without increasing what you eat. That amounts to ten pounds a year. . . . Or you could eat those extra calories, walk, and still maintain your present weight. Don't worry about exercise increasing your appetite. It won't . . . it may even decrease it."

Walking is part of most physical fitness programs for other sports. With just a bit of analytical thinking you can incorporate a walking program as part of your routine—walking to the stores, walking to your friend's home, walking to the bowling alley, walking at least part of the way to your office, walking the children home from school, driving on a weekend to an open area for a family walk, walking with your friend rather than stopping for a cocktail.

Not only will you be participating in a national energy conservation program, but your entire body will function better and you'll see around you architecture and foliage and people and sunsets that you never before noticed!

Chapter 14
When You Consult Your Podiatrist . . .

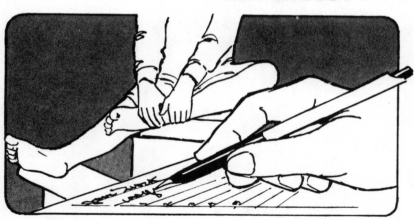

Now that you know how systemic conditions can affect your feet, you can readily understand why your podiatrist is interested in your complete physical history. Your past illnesses, current ailments for which you're under treatment, any operations you've ever had—all of these factors can help him to help you.

He is also concerned about your way of life. If you're a salesman, are you indoors standing behind a counter or are you outdoors walking and carrying a fifty pound valise? If you're a secretary, do you also keep house—including the marketing, cooking and ironing? If you're an executive, are you at your desk all day or do you spend much of the day going through a plant that has cement floors? If you're a teacher, do you stand or do you sit for most of the day?

What are your hobbies? Do you play tennis three times a week? Do you jog each morning? If you paint or sculpt, do you stand or sit as you work? Do you enjoy social dancing—and if not, why not?

What medications do you take? Do you take them on a specific schedule or just occasionally?

Some patients erect barriers to a good diagnosis.

One example is a reluctance to tell their age. Obviously a patient's age is important because certain problems develop more frequently in one age group than in another. Another barrier to good diagnosis is the attitude, "It's just a corn. Why is a whole history necessary?"

If the doctor can hurdle such psychological barriers, the patient is often surprised at how important his answers are! What he tells the doctor might explain that lower back pain at the end of the day. He may not know it, but that fracture of the right foot ten years ago might be related to the current problem on the left foot. His responses might establish the connection between that bunion that has increased in size and the corn that is now the reason for the consultation.

Your podiatrist will want a very specific history of any current injury or pain. When did the injury occur? Under what circumstances? How long have you had the pain? Did it start suddenly? Has it increased in severity? Is the pain constant? If not, when do you have pain? What is the nature of the discomfort—a sharp pain, a dull ache?

In examining you, your podiatrist will check for abnormalities in various areas such as bone structure, circulation, nerve supply, muscle power and gait.

One of his very important diagnostic tools is the x-ray. X-rays do not comprise a total examination, but they are often an indispensable part of a total examination.

I have found many surprises on x-rays, often in areas of which the patient was not complaining.

Vickie, a well-educated, apparently healthy young

192

woman of thirty-one, consulted me recently because of a pain in her great toe. In addition to the rest of the examination, I took x-rays.

I've read a lot of x-rays, but these made me stop short! There, unmistakably, was a sewing needle nestled between her fourth and fifth metatarsal bones. Even the eye of the needle was so well defined that it seemed to beg for a thread.

Vickie could offer no explanation. She was unaware of ever having stepped on a needle. In the operating room, where she had been given a local anaesthetic, she was amazed at the appearance of the needle, completely imbedded in decayed tissue and broken at the point where it had entered bone.

Obviously some conditions simply cannot be adequately diagnosed without x-rays.

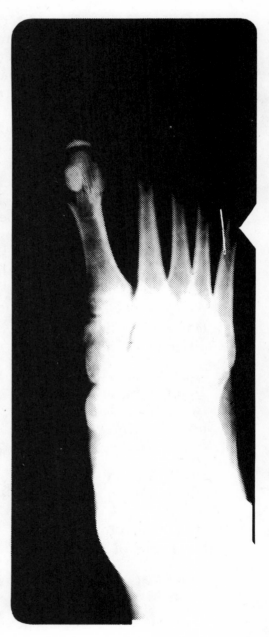

SOME "DON'T"S AND SOME "DO"S

Don't cut your corns or callus.

Do see your podiatrist on a time, not a pain, schedule. By the time you're in pain, you're in trouble. And why have unnecessary pain?

Don't use over-the-counter foot medications that are not prescribed.

Do call your podiatrist if any foot abrasion, rash or abnormality appears between your routine visits.

Don't soak your feet in hot water.

Do soak your feet in comfortably warm water if soaking is indicated.

Don't cut your nails with a scissor or nail cutter.

Do use an emery board on your nails—nothing else.

Don't allow the areas between your toes to remain wet for long periods of time.

Do remember always to dry thoroughly between your toes after bathing or swimming.

Don't use any abrasive material, such as a pumice stone or a file, on your heels or on any other part of your foot.

Do consult your podiatrist about any cracks in your heels and use a lubricant on your feet daily.

Don't tear or cut the skin between your toes.

Do ask your podiatrist about whatever abnormality you have between

194

your toes—a fissure (crack), a soft corn, a fungous infection or an ulcer.

Don't depend on medication to sedate cramps of your feet and legs.

Do have your podiatrist examine you to determine whether the cause of discomfort is in your walking posture.

Don't accept fatigue as a chronologic penalty.

Do check with your podiatrist to see whether faulty gait is not at least a contributing cause of your fatigue.

Don't use a heating pad or hot water bottle in bed.

Do wear bed socks, use additional blankets or keep the room temperature even by means of a thermostatically controlled electric heater.

Don't expect shoes to fit you if your feet elongate so that they jut all the way to the front of the shoes.

Do get professional advice before you buy your shoes.

Don't—don't—don't give up walking.

Do—do—do—walk, even if it's just a block at a time. Help your feet to help the rest of your body keep you active.

Glossary

Arteriosclerosis   a condition in which there is thickening, hardening, and loss of elasticity of the walls of blood vessels, especially arteries. It is commonly called hardening of the arteries.

Athletes foot   a non-medical term used to describe fungous infections. Fungous infections occur not only between the toes, on the sole of the foot and under the nails, but also on other parts of the body.

Ball of the foot   the front part of the foot, not including the toes. It is known more accurately as the metatarsal area.

Bromidrosis   a condition in which sweat has an offensive odor. It generally responds to treatment.

Buerger's disease *(thromboangiitis obliterans)*   a circulatory disease affecting chiefly the arteries and veins of the limbs. People with this disease require special care of the feet because of the decreased blood supply to the lower extremities.

Bunion   an enlargement of the joint behind the great toe. As the joint becomes increasingly deformed, not only the great toe, but other toes are pushed out of their proper position.

Callus   a thickening of the skin, developing in flat planes as a result of recurrent friction and pressure.

Club nail   a thickened, deformed nail. It often is caused by an injury to the nail. If it is not treated, it may become so thick that the pressure of the shoe on it causes pain.

Compound tincture of benzoin   a solution useful in the treatment of fissures. It can be bought without a prescription.

Congenital flatfoot   a foot with a flat arch at birth. This is a very serviceable foot, free of the arch problems so many people develop.

Cookie   a stiff material, concave in shape, for insertion in a shoe, supposedly to support the wearer's arch.

Corn   a circumscribed, cone-shaped thickening of the skin, that develops because of recurrent friction and pressure.

Diuretic   a medication to increase urination.

***Dorsalis pedis* pulse**   the pulse found on top of the foot. It is found on a line extending back from the space between the great toe and the second toe.

***Extensor brevis digitorum* muscle**   the only muscle with its origin on the top of the foot. It is found on the outer side of the top of the foot in front of the ankle.

197

Fissures   cracks in the skin, often between the toes or around the heels. Compound tincture of benzoin is sometimes prescribed for fissures, but, in many cases, other treatment is preferable.

Flatfoot (acquired)   a foot the arch of which becomes flat after birth.

Gait   the manner of walking.

Gastrocnemius **muscle**   the largest of the muscles in the back of the leg. It attaches to the heel by means of the tendo-Achilles.

Gout   one form of arthritis. The joint behind the great toe is an area frequently involved, but other areas may be affected. A high uric acid is associated with gout.

Hammertoe   a toe deformed in a flexed position. Since the toe is bent upward, the top of the shoe often irritates it, causing a corn. If the corn is neglected, an ulcer may develop.

Hematoma   a swelling containing blood.

Hyperhidrosis   a condition of excessive sweating that can be helped with treatment.

Ingrown nail   a nail impinged upon by the adjacent flesh. If it is not treated, an infection may develop.

Intermittent claudication   severe pain of leg muscles, during walking, but not when resting. The person with intermittent claudication can usually walk a specific distance, as three blocks, and then must rest. Eventually the distance decreases.

Lasting tacks   tacks used in shoe construction.

Lift (heel lift)   a piece of resistant material (as

198

leather, rubber or a synthetic) attached to the bottom of the heel of a shoe. A heel lift is approximately a quarter of an inch. One heel lift can be added to or taken off a shoe without affecting the tilt of the shoe.

Ligament a band of strong fibers connecting one bone to another.

Longitudinal arch the area extending from the heel to the ball on the inner side of the foot.

Mary Janes girl's strapped shoes, generally of patent leather. They are generally the "party" shoes of little girls.

Matrix of the nail the area from which the nail grows. It is not visible when looking at the nail plate.

Metatarsal area the area at the ball of the foot. The front ends of the metatarsal bones are found here. There is no real arch at the metatarsal area.

Metatarsal pad a pad put into the shoe or on the foot at the metatarsal area.

Nail bed the area visible through the attached portion of the nail.

Nail groove the space between the sides of the nail and the soft tissue. This is the area that becomes involved in an ingrown nail problem.

Onychomycosis a fungous infection of the nail. It is usually painless. It should be treated to avoid spread of the infection. It can often be recognized by yellowish streaks on the nail. A culture should be done, however, to verify the diagnosis.

Plantar verruca   a wart on the bottom of the foot. This term is used because the plantar surface of the foot is the bottom surface. *Verrucae* tend to increase in number and can become very painful. They should be treated.

Podiatrist   one who diagnoses and treats the disabilities, abnormalities and diseases of the feet.

Posterior tibial pulse   the pulse found behind the bone on the inner side of the ankle.

Pronation   the act of rolling to the inner side of the foot on weight bearing.

Proud flesh *(wilde Fleisch)*   a mass of excessive growth of painful soft tissue. On the foot it often develops in neglected ingrown nail problems.

Pseudo-sinus   a channel going into the flesh in an area of abnormality, such as in an ulcer.

Psoriasis   a skin disorder that sometimes affects the nails. It must be differentiated from *onychomycosis.*

Raynaud's Disease   a circulatory disease affecting the extremities, particularly in response to cold temperature. The hands, as well as the feet, are usually involved.

Reflexology (zone therapy)   a method of applying pressure to charted areas on the foot, supposedly to treat various parts of the body.

Scaphoid raise   a convex elevation, usually of hard rubber, for insertion in the shoe, supposedly to support the wearer's arch.

Sesamoid bones   small bones lodged in tendon.

	They are found in various parts of the body. The patella is an example.
Shoe-last	a wooden reproduction of the approximate shape of the human foot, over which a shoe is made.
Soleus **muscle**	one of the muscles in the back of the leg. Along with the gastrocnemius, it connects to the heel by the tendo-Achilles.
Sphincter	circular muscle constricting an opening, as of the bladder.
Spicule	a small, needle-shaped particle, as of nail or bone. Pain in a nail groove is often caused by spicules of nail left after attempts at self treatment.
Supernumerary bones	bones in addition to those usually found in the body. They may exist in various parts of the body.
Tendo-Achilles	the strongest, thickest tendon in the body. It connects the gastrocnemius muscle and soleus muscle.
Tendon	bands of strong fibers connecting muscle to bone or to other parts, such as another tendon.
Thromboangiitis obliterans **(Buerger's disease)**	a circulatory disease affecting chiefly the arteries and veins of the limbs. People with this disease require special care of the feet because of the decreased blood supply to the lower extremities.
Ulcer	a break in the continuity of tissue, leading to disintegration of the underlying tissue.
Verruca	a wart. Warts are benign tumors. They

require treatment, since they may increase in number. Verrucae can become very painful.

Wart a benign tumor, sometimes caused by a virus. It is also called a *verruca.*

***Wilde Fleisch* (proud flesh)** a mass of excessive growth of painful soft tissue.

Zone therapy (reflexology) a method of applying pressure to charted areas on the foot supposedly to treat various parts of the body.

Index